ENVELOPED LIVES

ENVELOPED LIVES

Caring and Relating in Lithuanian
Health Care

Rima Praspaliauskiene

CORNELL UNIVERSITY PRESS   ITHACA AND LONDON

First published 2022 by Cornell University Press

Library of Congress Cataloging-in-Publication Data

Names: Praspaliauskiene, Rima, author.
Title: Enveloped lives : caring and relating in Lithuanian health care
    / Rima Praspaliauskiene.
Description: Ithaca [New York] : Cornell University Press, 2022. | Includes
    bibliographical references and index.
Identifiers: LCCN 2022000659 (print) | LCCN 2022000660 (ebook) |
    ISBN 9781501765469 (hardcover) | ISBN 9781501766114 (paperback) |
    ISBN 9781501766077 (epub) | ISBN 9781501766084 (pdf)
Subjects: LCSH: Medical economics—Social aspects—Lithuania. | Medical
    economics—Moral and ethical aspects—Lithuania. | Medical care, Cost
    of—Social aspects—Lithuania. | Exchange—Social aspects—Lithuania. |
    Lithuania—Social conditions—1991–
Classification: LCC RA410.55.L58 P73 2022 (print) | LCC RA410.55.L58 (ebook) |
    DDC 338.4/73621—dc23/eng/20220124
LC record available at https://lccn.loc.gov/2022000659
LC ebook record available at https://lccn.loc.gov/2022000660

For Giedrius and Veronika

Contents

Preface

During my research and later when I presented my work, I was often asked about my experiences with money in public health care. Talking to my interlocutors and doing fieldwork at Vilnius Hospital revived my memories, so I begin this book with those.

I grew up in the Soviet Union and often visited my mom and aunt, who worked in hospitals. On the way to my mom's workplace, I would go through the small hospital park, passing patients sitting on benches and smoking cigarettes in their pajamas. I still remember the smell of chlorine and crisp, starched white coats, dim corridors painted dark green, rooms with missing tiles, and sun-lit nurse offices decorated with flowers. Snippets of the conversations about supply shortages, drunk patients, and practitioners still float in my memory. I also remember the slices of cake wrapped in paper napkins that my mother brought home for me. Hospital staff often shared the sweets that patients had given them.

Like the people I talked to, I hold memories of my enveloped encounters. I have an image of a big black smoked eel dripping with fat in my grandmother's hand. My uncle had given it to her, and he had received it as a present from one of his students. The smell of it filled the whole apartment. I remember badly wanting a slice of that eel. I was at home, released from the children's hospital for a weekend. I was five or six years old then. "I want that," I told my grandmother Veronika, who, unlike my mother, was much more inclined to grant my wishes. "No! This eel is for your doctor," my grandmother stated firmly. I was appalled by such a stupid idea. Why give this delicious eel to the woman who had ordered me those painful injections three times a day and kept me in the hospital? And she would get the whole eel! I hated the doctor who would deprive me of this delicacy. It was proof that life was not fair.

I soon learned that the boxes of chocolates in our buffet were also not for me. They were always meant for someone else: a dentist, a massage therapist, the nurse who gave me injections, the local librarian who set aside novels my mother loved, a saleswoman in a shoe store who would tell my mother when imported winter boots were due to arrive so that we could buy them before they sold out. These boxes of chocolates came and went from the buffet in the living room unless I disrupted their intended journey by opening them and sneaking a piece or an unexpected guest arrived and was offered them.

The same boxes of chocolates appeared in my friends' almost-identically furnished living rooms in our uniform apartment buildings. Sneaking chocolates from these boxes was a common temptation for kids. It was not hard to pull off the ribbon and open the box, take a candy or two, then rearrange the candies, close the box, and put the ribbon back on. My friends and I had almost perfected the art. Perhaps some of the boxes had been opened before I got to them, with a candy or two missing from the box. I do not know whether these boxes were marked or whether they ever held money, like in the stories everyone had heard. I never found anything but chocolates inside.

In the mid-1990s, my mother decided it was time for her to get surgery on her ruptured hernia. She had run into her surgeon on the street, and he told her that he was leaving for another city. He suggested my mother get the operation before he left. She told me about it when I was away at a conference, and I could only come back to take care of her on the day of the procedure. They had already operated on her when I entered the room that she was sharing with another woman. On the hospital bed, hooked up to IVs, my mother looked frail. I was sitting at her bedside when she started waking up from the anesthesia. She opened one eye and nodded. A few minutes later she tried to say something to me that I could not quite get. It seemed like she was asking me, "Did you thank the doctor?" I thought she was hallucinating. I had not seen the doctor. The nurses were checking in on her regularly, and they seemed friendly. She had already had the surgery. I had no idea I had to meet the doctor. After an hour or so she asked me again. I realized that she was serious. There was another patient in the room, and I felt ashamed. This whole conversation seemed inappropriate to me. My mother noticed that I was lost. "We talk," she said, referring to the other woman in the room, "her son already gave." Only then did I understand what she was referring to. I saw the disappointment on my mother's face. Like many of my interlocutors, I was not prepared for any of that.

I wrote this book to figure out how public health care and its medical culture, infused with seemingly unethical and corrupt practices like giving gifts and money to doctors, has carried on for so many decades of Soviet socialism and postsocialist capitalism. I wanted to understand how this configuration of care made sense for patients, their relatives, and doctors, and how the privatization and marketization of health care emerged as a dominant alternative to curtail it. At a time when health-care reforms and the costs of care are being debated widely, this book, even though it is written from a particular place—Lithuania—contributes to the larger debate about the ethics and futures of health care.

Acknowledgments

This book stems from care-full relations. They nurtured and carried me throughout the research and writing of this book. I am highly indebted to all who trusted me and shared their stories and practices and, like me, wanted to grasp the complexity of life and choices we make and the worlds that envelop us. This book would not have been possible without patients and their caregivers, doctors, nurses, state officials, and activists in Lithuania, who shared their experiences, allowed me to observe their work, and let me into their lives. I want to thank Transparency International Lithuania for sharing its materials and activities. I am grateful to the medical practitioners and the administration of a university hospital in Vilnius that I call "Vilnius Hospital" who granted me access, gave me their precious time, and were patient with me hanging around. You know who you are. I cannot name you, but I am highly indebted to you all.

My deepest gratitude goes to my advisers and mentors at the University of California, Davis. I could not wish for better guidance from the start to the end of this book. Their strong support, intellectual stimulation, and generous critiques carried me through all the rifts. First, I want to thank Joe Dumit, who taught me to read and think with texts. Joe's capacity to understand my book before I was able to see it clearly gave me strength. He made me think about capitalism in ways I had not imagined before. Joe's ability to attend to the particulars and play with ideas has always incited me. Marisol de la Cadena has been a continuous inspiration for my work. It was Marisol who encouraged me to do fieldwork in Lithuania and supported my passions. She showed me how to think through relations. Marisol's rigorous ethnographic thinking challenged me to be more complex and courageous. Cristiana Giordano inspired my interest in medical anthropology and was present at every stage of this work. She taught me to value the art of ethnographic writing, listening, and intellectual intrigue. Li Zhang has always been extremely supportive and provided generous space to think. Her knowledge of the postsocialist worlds, genuine concern, and commitment to clarity sharpened my thinking. Thank you all.

Friendships that began at UC Davis Anthropology Department fostered the intellectual project of this book. At UC Davis I learned from Tim Choy, Donald Dunham, Suad Joseph, Alan Klima, Rachel Parrenas, Suzana Sawyer, and many others. I was surrounded by a creative and caring collective—Jake Culbertson,

Bascom Guffin, Chris Kortright, Ingrid Lagos, Jieun Lee, Kristina Lyons, Lena Meari, Julia Morales, Tim Murphy, Melissa Salm, Camilo Sanz, Michelle Stewart, and Adrian Yen—that allowed me to grow intellectually. Sawyer seminar "Indigenous Cosmopolitics" at UC Davis was a gift of thinking together and a formative moment for my book.

I spent six months as a fellow at the Imre Kertesz Kolleg at the F. Schiller University in Jena among thinkers and experts of the twentieth-century culture and history of Eastern Europe: Slavka Ferencuchova, Agnieszka Jagòdzinska, Barbara Klich, Pawel Machcewicz, and Jan Mervart. The presence of Eva Clarita Pettai and Lars Fredrick Stocker at the Kolleg was a gift that gave me a rare opportunity to share my work and ideas with the scholars of the Baltic States. It was a bliss to discuss anthropology, history, and fate of Eastern Europe with Stefan Dorondel and Tomasz Rakowski. Natalia Aleksiun's optimism and encouragement gave me peace of mind. Special thanks to Joachim von Puttkamer and Michal Kopecek for welcoming me into the Kolleg community. Finally, Daniela Gruber, Diana Joseph, and Raphael Utz went above and beyond to create a supporting environment for the fellows. I am grateful for my time in Jena, Turingia.

Writing groups and writing partners were a vital part of my writing process. I am indebted to the Meds working group at the Center for Science Technology and Medicine at UC Berkeley, especially to Elena Conis, Sandra Eder, and Laura Nelson. I am grateful to Sonia Rab Alam, Heather Dron, Chris Hanssmann, and Krista Sigurdson for the supportive environment at UCSF.

"Smokies" with Jenna Grant and Marieke van Eijk kept me going when I thought it was impossible. "Muzu takas" helped me get through the finish line.

Parts of this book and its arguments were shared with and benefited from various audiences. SOYUZ Annual Symposiums at University of Michigan and Havinghurst Center, Miami University, Cascadia seminar "Adventures in Medical Anthropology" at the University of Washington, UC Davis Global Health Cluster, the Institute for the Study of Societal Issues and the Center for Science, Technology and Medicine at UC Berkeley, Miami University. In particular, I am grateful to Marianne de Laet, Eugene Raikhel, Michele Rivkin-Fish, Emily Yates-Doerr, and Alexei Yurchak for their comments.

I also greatly benefited from conversations with Maryna Bazylevych, Lawrence Cohen, Judith Farkuhar, Angela Garcia, Cori Hayden, Tomas Matza, Annemarie Mol, Tanya Richardson, Elisabeth F. Roberts, and Lisa Stevenson. Especially I want to thank Vincanne Adams for her insightful advice, feedback, patience, and support.

I am grateful to Anitra Grisales for her extraordinary guidance through the transformation of this book. I want to thank the editor at Cornell University Press, Jim Lance, for believing in this book. Mary Kate Murphy and Irina Burns helped to improve the manuscript. I want to thank Clare Jones, Brock Schnoke, and everyone else at Cornell University Press for their amazing work. I am also grateful to two anonymous reviewers for constructive feedback and encouragement.

The research and writing of this book would not have been possible without the support of the Anthropology Department at the University of California at Davis, the American Council of Learned Societies Fellowship in Eastern European Studies, Wenner-Gren Dissertation Fieldwork Grant and the Mellon-Sawyer fellowship, and Wenner-Gren Hunt Postdoctoral Fellowship.

Prior versions of some of the material in this book appeared in the following works: "Enveloped Lives: Practicing Health and Care in Lithuania," *Medical Anthropology Quarterly* 30, no. 4 (2016): 582–89 (Winner of the Steven Polgar Paper Prize); "La petite enveloppe au docteur ou la politique de la vie dans la Lituanie contemporaine," *Ethnologie Française* 48, no. 2 (2018): 297–304; "The Case of the Cake: Dilemmas of Giving and Taking," in *The Ethnographic Case*, ed. Emily Yates-Doerr and Christine Labuski (Mattering Press, 2018), https://www.matteringpress.org/books/the-ethnographic-case; and "Fieldnotes on Bribes, Smiles and Myths," *Anthropology News*, October 31, 2019, https://www.anthropology-news.org/articles/fieldnotes-on-bribes-smiles-and-myths/.

I feel blessed with my family of friends that surrounded me with love and care in both Lithuania and California. During the fieldwork my Lithuanian *familia*—longtime friends and companions—enveloped me with warmth and care, shared stories and meals, and their routines. Virginija Aleksejunė, Erika Grigoravičienė, Margarita Jankauskaitė, Laima Kreivyte and Santa Lingevičiute, Saulius and Ingrida Kvedaravičius, Vilana Pilinkaitė, Elena and Kazimieras Praspaliauskas, Loreta Raulinavičiūtė, Laisvyde Šalčiūtė, Gražina Sluckaite, JolitaValantiejiene, and Dagna Volkovaite—you made my fieldwork possible. I am grateful to Vida, Kastis, and Linas Chechavicius, Diana and Vidas Placiakis, Agne Sluckaite, and Solveiga Armoskaite for their friendship and patience with me. Your presence and sharing the worlds between Lithuania and the United States make my life and work attainable. Aiste Cechaviciute's presence, her laughter and energy during the pandemic and the last year of writing this book sustained me. Cristiana Giordano has been a nourishing friend, colleague, mentor, and an inseparable part of my family of friends. Thank you for being with me and caring for me beyond anthropological engagements.

I am indebted to my colleagues and friends, whose closeness I felt despite being separated by long distances. They were with me from the beginning of this book up until the end. I shared my joys and frustrations with anthropology and writing with Vivian Choi, Stefanie Graeter, and Zeynep Gursel. Jonathan Echeverri's ability to spark conversations and work collectively was a gift. Karina Vasilesvka-Das was a crucial interlocutor who read my work from medical anthropology and Baltic perspectives. I am grateful to Neringa Klumbyte for productive exchanges, her feedback, support, and comradery in writing this book. Fabiana Li was always there for me when I needed advice or help. My gratitude goes to Nicholas D'Avella for reading and commenting on many parts of this book and for being an attentive listener and thoughtful thinker. I cannot imagine this journey without Rossio Motta, her companionship and wit. I thank you all for sharing your thinking, laughter, the good and the bad.

I cannot find proper words to express my deepest gratitude and debt to Giedrius Praspaliauskas for his unconditional love, companionship, and support from the beginning to the end of this process, through ups and deep downs in making this book. I would not be here without you. This book is for you.

ENVELOPED LIVES

ENVELOPED CARE

After forty-five minutes of moving through the sleepy, snowy, and gray streets of the city in November 2009, a prerecorded female voice announced to the passengers on the bus: "The clinic: last stop." For the sick, the clinic is sometimes indeed the last stop on a journey through the maze of public health care that begins with the family doctor and may continue with visits to the local polyclinic, the regional hospital, or a private clinic. Patients are referred to this clinic in Vilnius, the capital of Lithuania, for complex diagnoses and advanced surgery.

The passengers—patients, nurses, relatives, doctors, students, and residents—stepped off the bus and dispersed, passing crowded parking lots and a line of kiosks that had sprung up in the city in the early 1990s, following independence from the Soviet Union. The kiosks, which are almost obsolete in other parts of Vilnius, sell necessities and treats for hospital patients, staff, and visitors: flowers, pajamas, slippers, deep-fried pastries, and a wide variety of chocolate bars and boxes. There is also a newsstand that carries newspapers and an abundant supply of white envelopes.

Inside the main entrance of the hospital there is another newsstand, a café, a pharmacy, and an ATM. That morning I tried to buy a little white envelope at the newsstand on the first floor of the clinic. It was not my first attempt. A middle-aged saleswoman wearing a sheepskin vest told me, as she had before, "Sorry, I am out of them; they go pretty fast. Try the kiosk outside, at the bus stop." When a woman behind me in line also asked for an envelope, the saleswoman said, "I am sorry, but you know what—just use a piece of regular white paper and fold it," and handed the woman a sheet of paper from the printer on her desk.

While I was still at the counter, caught by the scene, the saleswoman turned to me. "Miss, do you also need one? Take it, it will work," she said reassuringly.

What are these envelopes, and how do they work?

Little Envelopes

Vokelis (in Lithuanian), the little white envelope, epitomizes the relations of health care in contemporary Lithuania. Its function is to hold cash that patients or their families offer to doctors working in the public health-care system. These envelopes are variously described as "bribes," "gifts," "honoraria," "thank-yous," "informal payments," "additional," "nontransparent," and "nontaxable income."[1] Often they are placed in gift bags that might also contain boxes of chocolates, bottles of alcohol, or postcards. Although this practice of informal payments to doctors is ubiquitous, it is also contested. Some patients and their caregivers said they felt no qualms about giving thank-you payments, while others condemned the doctors who accepted them as greedy. Doctors talked about their conflicted feelings of gratitude for and dependence on patients' alms and their obligations to their families. Almost everyone was caught up in these dilemmas.

These informal payments are a distinctive element of medical culture in Eastern Europe and other postsocialist contexts. They have been linked to the scarcity of resources in socialist economies and to the turbulent transitions to capitalism, both working against and sustaining the socialist state. In 2009 and 2010, I was doing research during health-care reform led by the Ministry of Health of Lithuania. The reform project (2008–18) focused on hospital optimization and aimed to transform the practice of informal payments for medical treatment into a system of official copayments.[2] Transparency International Lithuania (TIL), the local branch of a global nongovernmental organization that exposes corruption in government and business transactions, had organized seminars and produced visual materials urging Lithuanians not to engage in what it called bribery.[3] State officials, however, were reluctant to blame doctors or accuse them of accepting bribes and were ambivalent about the privatization of public health care. Managers of private health-care clinics and experts from the Free Market Institute (Laisvosios rinkos institutas), a neoliberal think-tank, complained extensively in the local media that informal payments, "the culture of envelopes," were significantly impeding the transformation of public health care from a social function of the state to a business matter.

Envelopes were being blamed for the failure to develop viable private health insurance policies and standards that could effectively demarcate and organize patients according to their health insurance cards. Thus, they were characterized as an obstacle to the growth of private medical services. Policymakers, international and local experts, and scholars represented the shift from informal to official payments as more ethical, lawful, and moral. According to many of the free-market proponents, this transformation would also open fair competition between public and private health-care institutions and provide more choices to health-care consumers. If money changed hands, it had to be on the open market, they said. Otherwise, the health-care system would be stuck in the Soviet past, burdening the state with too many financial obligations. This characterization of the envelope as an obstacle to both the privatization of health care and the survival of public institutions intrigued me. Over the course of my research, I came to understand it as so much more.

This book examines the envelope as an ethnographic concept through the notion of relations, complicating the distinction between gifts and bribes, money and payment, transparency and corruption. I perceive ethnography as a concept-making genre and its concepts as "concrete abstractions" (de la Cadena and Blaser 2018). The envelope as a concept emerged from my fieldwork in Lithuania from 2009 to 2010. In this book, it is simultaneously concrete and abstract. The envelope is a situated relation that allows me to follow and describe practices of care. It is a container for complex, moral doctor-patient-caregiver transactions—a nexus of relations. When opened, it reveals the ethics of care, the economy of relationships, and the political economy of health at the intersection of neoliberal reforms and the fragmentation of socialism. It thus epitomizes the contention between different ethical, political, and economic regimes.

This relational practice—what I call "enveloped care"—is configured through the interactions between people, stories, rumors, affect, money, and other material objects that patients and their caregivers offer to doctors. These items alter the market logic of exchange and interrupt the relation between service provider and customer. As patients are being transformed into customers through the introduction of fees for elective procedures, the persistent practice of enveloped care invokes the ongoing desire to be perceived not only as a patient but as a person and sometimes even to be treated as kin. It is thus embedded in complex social relations driven by webs of obligation that include both gratitude and the pressure to give. As this book shows, enveloped care operates through conflicting notions of care, treatment, and neglect. The relations it mediates are characterized by asymmetry, vulnerability, and dependency. Yet this practice can provide recognition and the potential for care in uncaring conditions. Enveloped care exposes the gaps in institutionalized medicine and, in some ways, fills them.

Anthropologists have examined the bribe-gift opposition, discussing questions of recognition and misrecognition, and the monetization of exchanges in informal relations (Humphrey 2002, 2012; Jasarevic 2016; Kornai 2001; Ledeneva

1998; Patico 2002; Rivkin-Fish 2005, 2011). Some argue that neoliberal reforms in Eastern Europe have intensified the predatory side of monetary offerings to doctors, turning them into payments and thus succumbing to market forces (Stan 2012). But in my observations, the envelope exceeds the notions of a gift or a bribe, while also being included in them. Instead of elaborating on the gift-bribe or gift-commodity foil or focusing solely on the material transaction itself, I examine the ambiguous relations and ambivalent practices that constitute this informal practice. These dynamics go beyond economic rationality and thus allow it to persist.

I view the envelope as a precapitalist economic form and a site to rethink the "unquestioned authority of capitalism in our lives" (Tsing 2015, 65). Often considered a remnant of socialism, the envelope is surviving amid market capitalism. It remains an integral and vexing part of the Lithuanian healthscape.[4] This book, then, looks at why this precapitalist economic form is still thriving and what it might mean for ongoing neoliberal reforms. I argue that one key to its survival is that the envelope is both a vehicle for and an expression of what I refer to as the "will to care."[5] In the Lithuanian context, the will to care is a manifestation of the personal or collective attempt to preserve life and relationships in the face of illness and the shifting political economy of health. It both pushes back on the limitations of the health-care system, whether socialist or market-based, and demands recognition of a patient's singularity. This will to care emerges from kin obligations to take care of family members, friends, and relationships at all costs, forging what I call "caring collectives." This collective care gives people the sense that they have more of a grip on medical encounters and illness. In this context, the envelope is a collective explanatory site for patients and caretakers to interpret medical encounters, illness prospects, and potential outcomes. The envelope thus is built on and facilitates relationships between doctors and patients and between patients and their families, while also being an incarnation and practice of care.

It's Personal

"I don't know about you, but for me the little envelope is an emotional contact (*vokelis—tai jausminis kontaktas*). It saved my life." Lucija, a fifty-four-year-old copy editor of a cultural magazine, told me this when we sat down to talk at a café in Vilnius. She had given quite a few little envelopes to doctors in the public health-care system, and I was a bit surprised that Lucija started our conversation with such a firm, positive statement about envelopes. Knowing that she was skillful and careful with words, I realized that Lucija had thought about our conversation beforehand and wanted to define her position. Her opening sentence contrasted sharply with Transparency International's narratives of corruption and the definition of all informal material or monetary transactions between patients (or their families) and doctors as bribes. Lucija's explanation of how the envelope was an affective transaction that saved her life shaped my inquiry into the informal economy of illness.[6]

I had run into Lucija two days before, at a bus stop on a breezy November afternoon in 2009. I was on my way to the TIL office, located in the old part of town in a building owned by George Soros. I had just returned to Lithuania, my home country, after eight years living abroad, to conduct my dissertation research. Suddenly, a woman walking by stopped, turned to me, and asked: "Rima? Do you remember me?" After a moment I recognized her voice and remembered her thin, metallic, oval eyeglasses. We had chatted occasionally back when I lived in Lithuania. Her appearance startled me: the plump and round-faced Lucija I had known ten years ago was half the size I remembered. When I asked her how she was doing, Lucija answered that it was a long story, not for an encounter at the bus stop. She inquired what I was up to. I told her briefly that I was studying informal payments that patients gave to doctors, and I was interested in healthcare reform in Lithuania, including the envelope system. I asked her whether she had spotted any posters asking patients not to bribe or signs with crossed-out envelopes. She had not seen any. When the bus arrived, we got on and continued our conversation. "I can be your subject," she told me, "I have spent more time in hospitals and polyclinics than in the editorial room in the last five years. I even thought about writing down everything that I have been going through. I will tell you. Call me." I called her the next day.

Lucija told me that after falling sick with a rare intestinal disease, she had undergone three years of treatment without any significant improvement. She was among 2 percent of patients with this disease who did not respond to medications. When Lucija was facing complicated surgery (doctors gave her a 20 percent chance of survival) and her world was collapsing, she made a bet with herself: if her doctor accepted the envelope, she would get better, but if he refused it, she would die soon. The envelope gave her hope.

Lucija was already familiar with the practice of giving money or food to doctors. She had given envelopes before and shared her experiences with friends, relatives, and colleagues. Now she was an expert. "I thought I was buying doctors, their service," she reflected on her past experiences. Like many patients and their family members, Lucija was ambivalent about giving envelopes. Some patients described this practice to me as "something you cannot escape," an "organic part of life," and a "cult of giving." Some said they had "no moral hesitation" in giving envelopes, whereas others felt pressured by greedy doctors or argued that patients were "spoiling" doctors in trying to procure exceptional care for themselves. Almost everybody agreed that the state was not spending enough on health care and doctors' salaries, even though they noticed improvements in medical technology and hospital facilities. Only a few supported an increase in taxes to fund health-care services for the rapidly aging population.

Giving envelopes to doctors, along with sharing illness experiences, was a common topic of conversation among families, friends, neighbors, coworkers, and in the media. I was even referred to a website where patients informally ranked doctors. The appropriate size of the gift was included in the questionnaire and displayed on the website.[7] Even those people who otherwise strongly opposed corrupt practices and supported policies of transparency made an exception when they or their family members faced illness. According to them, doctors were the only professionals who were "worthy" of envelopes because they "worked hard." Alternately, some felt provoked (*provokuoti, provokuoja*)—that is, urged to act in a certain way through verbal or nonverbal signals from doctors or nurses—while others said they gave money in response to pressure from fellow patients, friends, or family members. When doctors found themselves in the role of patients or caregivers, they too struggled with questions of whether and how much to give. Envelopes were a lens through which patients and caregivers tried to interpret or make sense of medical encounters.

When faced with serious illness, people often changed their positions from being against the envelopes to using and believing in them. Lucija vividly described how her perception had changed once she had pinned her hopes on the envelope she presented to her doctor. When the surgeon seemed hesitant to accept the envelope, Lucija started crying. Then the doctor took her envelope, which held 100 litai.[8] "It gave me hope that I would get better. . . . I think it is inhumane for doctors not to take money from patients who are giving them envelopes, even if they have terminal cancer and are going to die soon." As she spoke, she reached for a napkin to wipe away her tears. "They must take the money, and then, if they want to or they feel bad, they can return it to the families if the patient dies or when there really is no chance," she said passionately. For Lucija, the envelope was related to her belief in the future. She perceived the medical encounter as a pendulum swinging between life and death. The envelope could stabilize anxieties and uncertainties; it was a force that could keep death at bay, even if only temporarily. It became part of the treatment and healing process itself.

Medical clinical care, with its objective and impersonal scientific approach, often rubs up against local practices, patient experiences, and plural healing systems, as Lucija's story and many others in this book illustrate. Care is always ambiguous and local (Mol 2010). On the level of the individual, it seeks to maintain life in ways that are not necessarily rational or just, yet it still has collective effects. The envelope is a site of friction between this bioscientific, universal notion of health, and care as a particular lived experience—in other words, between biological and biographical notions of life.[9] Health metrics offer standardized conceptualizations of health, disease, the value of care, and the best payment options (Adams 2016). They measure the biological. In this book I focus on a different tool. I consider envelopes to be affective (bio)metrics based on the singularity of each patient and the notion of biographical life, things that institutionalized, depersonalized measures of health and care tend to leave out.

Filling the Gaps

Envelopes are situated in distinctive historical relationships between the state, medical practice, and the population. Knowing how to navigate them has been key to survival in Lithuania and Eastern Europe more broadly. Political and economic instability—including wars, occupations, upheavals, deportations, and shortages—are inscribed in the bodies, relationships, and practices of the region, including that of health care. Cultivating relationships and solidarities has been crucial to personal and family stability and well-being, whether during czarist rule, Soviet socialism, or during the three decades of neoliberal reforms that started in the 1990s.

In Lithuania, enveloped care dates back to and beyond the socialist state. After the Polish-Lithuanian Commonwealth was annexed and partitioned by Russia, Prussia, and Austria-Hungary in 1795, the health-care system in Lithuania was subjected to Russian laws. The imperial Russian state paid doctors' salaries through local districts (*zemstvos*), and patients were charged for treatment on a sliding scale (Bazylevych 2009; Keshavjee 2014; Knauss 1980). The amounts were left up to the doctors and patients to decide. According to a physician who practiced medicine before the Russian Revolution in 1917, "After treatment a patient would put in the doctor's hand whatever she felt the doctor deserved" (Knauss 1980, 71).

Lithuania became an independent republic in 1918, after World War I. Little is known about the health-care system during the interwar period of 1918–40. The majority of the population—farmers and agricultural workers—was not covered by health insurance (Norkus 2008; Pivorienė and Mikalauskaitė 2005). Villagers paid for doctors' visits with cash and food. Following the Soviet occupation of Lithuania in 1940, which was interrupted by the German occupation of 1941–44, treatment through the new state-run health-care system was officially free. Private medical practices were outlawed. The Soviet government struggled to eradicate any exchange of money and goods between patients and doctors, denouncing them as "bourgeois habits." Most of the patients ignored it (Vaiseta 2015, 54–55). Goods, money, and favors were present in medical encounters during socialism. Some people I talked to recalled that it was customary to give quite large amounts of money to doctors (10–25 rubles, compared to their salaries of 120 rubles).

In 1990, Lithuania became the first republic to break away from the Soviet Union and regained its sovereignty after fifty years of occupation. In 1995, Lithuania, along with other Baltic and Eastern European countries, applied to become a member of the European Union (EU). In 2000, the country started accession talks; after four years of negotiations, adjustments, and reforms, Lithuania's request was granted. At that time, the country enrolled in what Dace Dzenovska (2018, 89) calls "the school of Europeanness," rapidly learning "Western practices." Enveloped practices became a sign of backwardness, inherited from the Soviet past, and the epitome of corruption that had to end. The continued prevalence of enveloped practices held Lithuania in an uneasy place between the corrupt past and the transparent future of the EU.

After the fall of the Iron Curtain, massive changes swept through the newly independent states of the Soviet bloc. International lending agencies, public health researchers, and other experts anticipated that market economics would transform medical treatment into a consumer service through deregulation, decentralization, and rationalization (Bazylevych 2009; Koch 2013; Phillips 2011; Rivkin-Fish 2005). However, the informal economy did not disappear along with state socialism. In the words of Janos Kornai (2001), what had been "market socialism" became "a relic of socialism" that was surviving in a capitalist market economy and threatening the implementation of neoliberal health-care reforms. The process of transformation is not a simple replacement of the Soviet moral economy with immoral market mechanisms (Burawoy and Verdery 1999; Collier 2005, 2012; Dunn 2004; Foucault 1990, 2008; Hann 2002; Humphrey 2002; Ong and Rose 1999; Verdery 1996; Yurchak 2006; Zhang 2008). Enveloped practices of care reveal how the social is articulated at the core of complex ethical conditions in which socialist, postsocialist, and neoliberal regimes coexist in society at large and in medical settings

The socialist state was never able to regulate enveloped practices, which were left to partial self-governance. Patients and their caregivers have mastered enveloped practices as a form of self-cultivation, what Michel Foucault (1988) calls the "art of existence," which shapes certain modes of knowledge and care. By reproducing and refining enveloped practices, patients and caretakers find ways to obtain better health care, becoming experts of an informal economy of illness. It is customary to judge the health care of the population using metrics and indicators for health care outcomes, such as life expectancy, infant mortality, number of doctors, or the quality of technical infrastructure. That is how good health care is defined. As life expectancy in Lithuania began rising steadily in 1994, and millions were spent on upgrading hospitals and outpatient clinics, patients kept looking for better care. That category is not limited to successful surgeries, impressive laboratories, or diagnostic apparatuses. There is no doubt that new surgery rooms and diagnostic tools saved lives. Neurosurgeons and cardio surgeons "did wonders," patients acknowledged. But that was also not enough. Patients and caregivers often valued the medical care they received based on affective (bio)metrics—a measure of the singular experience of being cared for. How patients chose to reward doctors with envelopes and under which circumstances communicated how they measured that value. This was also the case with doctors' decisions from whom to accept envelopes and other gifts.

The Will to Care, for Oneself and Others

Not all envelopes exerted the same power as a pendulum between death and life, as had been the case for Lucija on the eve of her life-threatening surgery. When she had started seeing a gastroenterologist at the local polyclinic, Lucija decided to give her an envelope because "everybody did." She liked the doctor, whom she had to see quite often. After a few visits, Lucija wanted to give another envelope. The doctor refused, saying that Lucija already had a lot of expenses. Like many working in the cultural and educational fields, Lucija had a modest income, and she had spent a lot of money on copayments for medications and the restricted diet she had to follow. The next time Lucija saw the doctor, she brought her flowers. "I bought a big bouquet for the amount I wanted to give her—50 litai. When she said that to me about expenses, I felt that I wanted to thank her. She was honest and compassionate, and I felt close to her."

Afterward, however, Lucija decided that flowers were not a good idea. "I thought how silly it was to give her flowers. Maybe I was giving her flowers when she needed a facial cream, haircut, or a book, or she wanted to go to the opera or out to dinner at a restaurant." So, she switched back to giving the doctor envelopes with money. Although Lucija did not describe the doctor as her friend, whose preferences and concerns she was familiar with, she did emphasize the friendliness of the medical encounters. For the past three years she had been giving envelopes to her doctor twice a year: "one for Christmas and another one in the summer."

When I asked Lucija how she felt about "buying doctors," she answered, "Yes, I 'buy' a doctor, but that is how I feel safe." Then, she paused for a minute or two, looked out the window of the café, and said: "In a way we buy family members and friends too. It is the same with doctors. Each time I give her money, I feel more connected to this gastroenterologist." Her remarks evoke the long tradition in the anthropology of studying how gifts and debts make relations and persons (Godbout and Caille; Graeber 2010; Mauss 2000; Strathern 1990). Lucija trusts her doctor, who, according to her, would give her the right number of tests and prescriptions. She cares for herself, but she also cares for the doctor, "the good doctor," in a way she cares for other relationships. Money and caring are interwoven for Lucija. The ability of money to transform into objects, food, or experiences allows envelopes with money to be very personal while retaining a depersonalized appearance.

Studying the relation between caring and money has been on the fringes of medical anthropology. Although the current debates on care challenge assumptions of universality and reveal the complexities of medical care, the links between money, health, and care are just beginning to enter the discussion (see Jasarevic 2016; Roberts 2012). Scholars show how care is relational (Giordano 2014; Han 2012; Mol, 2010) and is expressed in careful engagements with words and gestures (Cohen 2008); it is a moral practice that makes caregivers (Kleinman 2009) and constitutes a process of voluntary affiliation (Borneman 1997). In other words, care is not "a category within defined borders," but a problem of everyday life (Han 2012, 23) and precarity (Matza 2018); it can be ambivalent and violent (Garcia 2010). The messiness of care that is ingrained in its ambivalence produces specific forms of care (Stevenson 2014). Doctor-patient relationships and monetary transactions are often treated as separate, unrelated spheres where care and exchange do not go together (Kleinman 1988; Mol 2010). However, comparatively little attention has been given to how the forms and practices of care are implicated in monetary relations, and how these relations mediate relationships between doctors, patients, and caregivers. Enveloped care can help us to understand these nuances.

"I appreciate when doctors don't play games, 'Oh, no, there is no need,' and I have to convince them to take an envelope. When they don't accept the money, it just distracts me. I don't want to be dismissed. Actually, when my envelope is refused, I feel spiritual discomfort (*dvasinis diskomfortas*). I know what I am doing," Lucija asserted. She did not seem to feel that the doctors were taking advantage of her. She wanted her decision to give to be accepted and recognized. What she emphasized was her agency during medical encounters. The envelope that Lucija was giving was a part of herself. It was not the act of giving, engaging in an ambiguous transaction, that caused her discomfort. It was the doctor's refusal that injured her.

The care of oneself, Foucault suggests, is a principle of self-cultivation that "presides over its development, and organizes its practices" (1988, 43). In

Lithuania, enveloped care likewise became what Foucault describes, in relation to taking care of one's body and health, as "a form of attitude, a mode of behavior; it became instilled in ways of living; it evolved into procedures, practices and formulas that people reflected on, developed, perfected and thought. It thus came to constitute a social practice, giving rise to relationships between individuals, to exchanges and communications, and at times even to institutions" (1988, 45). People reflect on the phenomenon of envelopes and tailor their behaviors and modes of communication accordingly. Enveloped care organizes relationships of doctors, patients, and caretakers, and these relationships, in turn, exert an effect on institutions. It is a way to maintain stability and quality of life in the face of shifting political and economic regimes; this drives the will to care for oneself and others.

Here I am building on Joao Biehl's concept of *the will to live*. Working in a community of AIDS survivors in Brazil, Biehl observed how residents refused to be overpowered by the forces of the neoliberal government and pharmaceutical companies that threatened their autonomy. This refusal, according to Biehl (2007, 400), is the immanence of life. The will to live is "a human force that is capable of acquiring sufficient consistency for turning a situation around—call it a language of hope—and transforms into a map of the present world: a broken world, full of rifts that deepen, yet also a world of previously unimaginable possibilities" (Biehl 2007, 405). This will to live refigures the terms of care and citizenship, articulated at the intersection of abandonment, medicine, and makeshift care, yet it is still an individualized form of care (Biehl 2007, 48–49, 308). I extend this from the personal will to live to the collective will to care. Like the will to live, the will to care also expresses a language of hope, as Lucija's case shows, but it underscores collective care for oneself and others. It is not limited to the survival of the individual because it is inseparable from collective obligations.

In going beyond the care of the self, enveloped care involves caring for others who need treatment—a family member, friend, neighbor, or relative—and the doctor or nurse who provides the treatment. In other words, care for one's self also entails a form of caring for the other that generates circuits of care, what I call "caring collectives," that emerge depending on the situation. This type of care has been criticized as a self-interested form that simply extends familial care and paternalistic notions to the public realm and thus does not lead to systemic change (Rivkin-Fish 2005). Joan C. Tronto (1993) sees this type of care as parochial and dangerous. According to Miriam Ticktin (2011), a politics of care that does not generate radical critique and preserves an existing order is antipolitics. I argue that even though enveloped care preserves the existing order and does not alleviate inequalities, it does interrupt the marketization and privatization of public health care in Lithuania.

In addition, enveloped care inverts the relations of caring by turning patients, traditionally conceived as objects of care, into agents of care who offer recognition, consideration, and generosity to medical practitioners. The patients I spoke with often expressed care for and solidarity with the doctors, commenting that the state does not adequately recognize doctors' work. This form of care is grounded in complex embedded relationships and affects the way health care is practiced in Lithuania. To frame the envelope as merely a form of corruption, a gratuity, a de facto fee for service, or a bribe fails to capture the complexities and contradictions of the phenomenon. Enveloped practices of care unfold to magical elements, generate hope and disappointment, and collapse ethical regimes. Examining these nuances allows us to shift the focus toward different ethics of care and different economy of relationships in the context of health care today.

Contested Values

"Wouldn't it be easier if there were no envelopes, and people could pay officially?" I asked Lucija. I wanted to know her views on the attempts to replace the envelope system with official copayments for medical visits. Numerous campaigns organized by TIL attempted to educate Lithuanian citizens "to not bribe" doctors and to not "participate in the culture of corruption," rather to embrace the Western values of liberal capitalism. The failures of Lithuania's health-care system have been explained through the idioms of transparency and corruption, too.[10] Thus, the policies of transparency are imagined as guarantors of better care. It is impossible to disagree that envelope practices are ambiguous; they do cause anxiety and can be experienced as harmful to both patients and doctors. There is a real danger that vulnerable patients are being taken advantage of and that these enveloped encounters lack dignity. Yet, as Lucija and many other people illustrated, these practices of giving also express gratitude and give pleasure. In this context, public health-care institutions are the sites of both mistrust and appreciation; they, too, embody ambivalence (Whitmarsh 2014).

Lucija was skeptical: "I like it as is, and I don't want official payments. This system comes from this society, and that is why it works so well. Even if you don't pay, you will get your surgeries done, and most likely nothing bad will happen to you. But if I value my life, I give, I feel better. I recognize this communication system and these relationships. It is safer for me. It is an unwritten deal (*toks nerašytas sandėris*) that each person can give according to his or her means. That is how it works. It is the only viable system (*vienintelė gyvybiška sistema*) because it is personal and concrete."[11]

Lucija also expressed concern that copayments, unlike envelopes, would disappear in "a big pot" with no certainty that her doctor would get the money. Lucija did not associate official payments with transparency or the systematic distribution of funds. She worried that her money would go to the administration to underwrite their expensive cars and more bureaucracy. "I want my doctor to get my money," she explained bluntly.

Is this kind of unwritten deal between patients, their family members, and medical practitioners a deal against the state, society, and capital? When the practice is ubiquitous, and a significant part of society is involved, whose interests does it work for and against? What values and ways of life is Lucija talking about? Andrea Ballestero refers to transparency as "a form of intervention into a world constituted by relations that can be molded, corrected, and regimented" (Ballestero 2012, 160). Lucija questioned this view. She did not see her experience framed by the ethics endorsed by TIL or the discourses of good governance (Webb 2012). In this context, transparency and care are not valued in the same way.

The envelope system, "the only viable system," in Lucija's estimation, has evolved within this society, with all its faults and contradictions, into its own system of relationships and communications. Lucija knows how to conduct these relationships. Maybe she is stuck in the past, as some would say. However, for Lucija, the envelope of money represents more than an economic transaction. Lucija emphasized that the practice of envelopes entails "giving according to a person's means." Not all patients give envelopes, and not all doctors accept them. The offerings in the envelopes may range from a chocolate bar to several hundred litai (or euros). The amount offered is carefully calculated according to the patient's diagnosis, financial means, familial negotiations, the doctor's attitude, and other affective (bio)metrics. In other words, there is no single principle that underpins the workings of the envelope.

Lucija is also deeply concerned about the fairness of official payments. How would they be distributed? Would they reward her doctor in the way she wants? Would they be fair to the doctors? Who will benefit from the new system? Most of the patients I talked to, whether they were comfortable with the envelopes or not, were opposed to official copayments. They wanted unlimited access to health care, free of charge.

By contrast, some doctors I talked to, particularly younger ones, had a positive view of privatization and official payments; they hoped to earn more if the practice changed. When I asked them what would happen to people who could not afford copayments or supplemental health insurance, I was told that such patients could go to "charity hospitals." In other words, these doctors imagined separate hospitals for different socioeconomic groups. Alternately, I also talked to some doctors who switched back from private clinics to public polyclinics because they did not want "to sell health." They felt the administrators were forcing them to generate income by prescribing more tests and referrals to specialized doctors. From their perspective, the future and success of market reforms did not seem so bright, despite being transparent and legal. The debates over the future of health care are not just about eliminating envelopes by instituting more sensible arrangements. They are not restricted to the eradication of "corruption."[12] The emphasis on transparency is crucial to understanding the rifts in neoliberal configurations of public health care. It entails a shift in the logic of the gift toward the logic of discrete payments and markets.

But what is transparency? Can envelopes be transparent? Envelopes are concealed transactions, and transparency is concerned with unveiling them and making them accountable. It is about the elimination of ambivalence. Phenomena become visible through the practices of description (Strathern 2000b, 312), and these descriptions also reveal details that can be viewed as data and information. For instance, in this book, the envelope is visible through the stories of interactions between patients and their relatives, doctors, and nurses. However, narratives about envelopes are individual and contextual. They resist objective analysis. These narratives cannot be easily translated into data, broken into equal units, or made uniformly applicable. As Byung Chul Han (2015) observes, things become transparent when they are integrated into the smooth streams of capital, communication, and information when they abandon their singularity and find expression through their price alone. Money in the envelope would become transparent via its transformation into a copayment that is accounted for and taxable.

This transformation would not eliminate the exchange of money in healthcare transactions or produce a return to free health care. Instead, transparency aims to replace the individual relation (thought to be embedded in the structures of inequality, political economy, and power) between the doctor and the patient with a somewhat organizational relation between the customer and health-care provider; the arrangement shifts from negotiated and open-ended to fixed and formalized. Care becomes a commodity, divisible into accountable units. Paradoxically, transparency also obscures facts about the nature of care being provided: issues of accessibility, trust and intimacy, social inequality, appropriation of the payments by capital, and commodification of doctor-patient relationships. In other words, a personal relationship is replaced with an impersonal transaction, part of an economy that Katherine Verdery describes as "a separate domain and a force of nature, for which no one in particular is responsible" (1996, 181).

The way patients and relatives assign value to envelopes is based on affective-(bio)metrics; these biographical and contextual calibrations make each envelope unique. This valuation differs from the numerical value of envelopes indexed by TIL's "corruption maps" or surveys commissioned by the state.[13] These surveys produce metrics that measure the level of corruption. The numbers show what percentage of patients gave money, how much, and even come up with the prices—or bribes—for each procedure, be it surgery, anesthesiology, or doctor's visit. These metrics are then popularized in the media. Their point is to show negative value—how much value is lost or hidden from the state—and evaluate the loss in monetary terms. The amounts of money passed from the patients to the doctors' pockets are considered as not only negatively impacting the state budget but also the growth and development of the health-care market. The only way to make up for this loss of value is to make envelopes transparent by turning them into copayments that are legal and thus ethical. However, losing a market does not necessarily mean that the value or care that patients attribute to doctors is lost. On the one hand, enveloped practices produce positive value (they are therapeutic and affective). On the other, envelopes have negative value (leading to economic loss and impeding market-based health-care reforms). They are valued by applying different systems—numerical and affective—that are in constant friction with what counts as desirable and good care.

An envelope of money given to a doctor transcends the material patient-doctor transaction itself and instead emerges as a productive force for coping with illness, medical encounters, and misfortunes. Enveloped care might appear individualistic, but it is not only limited to the relationship between individuals. In fact, interruptions in neoliberal health-care policies could end up being beneficial for patients. Envelopes do not reduce social inequality, but they have slowed down significantly the transformation of public health care from a social function of the state to a business matter, possibly precluding the emergence of new inequalities that could arise with the adoption of private health care and insurance regimes.

Opening the Envelope

After living abroad for eight years, in 2009 I went to Lithuania to conduct my dissertation research. The country was suffering from the effects of the 2008 financial crisis, but the government and the media avoided using the word "crisis." They believed that the linguistic choice directly affected reality. Instead, everyone was talking about "hard times" (*sunkmetis*). Austerity measures, such as the internal devaluation of litai, the local currency, slashed salaries in the public sector and pensions. Unemployment rose. My friends' belief in progress and free markets was shaken. Until then, it had seemed like the turmoil of the economic transformations of the first decade of independence from the Soviet Union were behind them. Lithuania had been on the path to prosperity, caching up with Europe, when the crisis hit.

Since Lithuania became a member of the EU in 2004, there was an influx of funding to integrate newly accepted members. Thousands of public servants went to other EU countries through exchange programs to learn best practices. Many more took advantage of the disappearance of borders and cheap flights to travel as tourists. University students took advantage of exchange programs and studied abroad. People smiled more. Cars honked less and stopped at intersections to let pedestrians cross the street without having to run. "Funded by the EU" signs were visible throughout Lithuania. Between 2004 and 2013, the health-care system alone received over 1.5 billion euros from the EU.[14] Every time I came back, I saw new shopping malls, apartment buildings, and newly renovated schools, hospitals, and roads. Vilnius's old town sprawled with cafes and tourists. Despite the shiny new exterior, not everyone was benefiting from the new prosperity. Inequality was steadily creeping up. Some of my friends were doing quite well, while others were struggling to make ends meet. Some had already left the country.

The financial crisis of 2008 was the impetus for a new wave of migration to the EU, significantly increasing the numbers of Lithuanians living and working abroad. This was similar to the previous wave of emigration that began when Lithuania became an EU member. Almost every family had somebody living in Britain, Ireland, or Norway. Migrants often came back for medical treatments. They also sent money to their relatives. Some of that money was offered in envelopes to medical practitioners. No matter how successful or unfortunate Lithuanians were, they all dealt with envelopes in the health-care system.

Inspired by the works of anthropologists who follow objects through their enactments in practice and by the analytics of partial connections (Mol 2002; Strathern 1991), I began tracing the field of relations that converged in those envelopes. During eighteen months of fieldwork, I conducted research at a hospital in Vilnius that I will call Vilnius Hospital, engaging in participant observation in four of the hospital's units: cardiology, surgery, mental health, and emergency.[15] I presented myself as an anthropologist studying health-care reform and practices. I tried to make clear my interest in the privatization of public health care and the transformation of the envelope system into transparent copayments. I showed my interview questions, including the ones about envelopes, to the hospital administration. Because I wanted to see how envelopes came up in conversations and medical settings, I often waited for the envelopes to be invoked or offered in my presence.

I sat in waiting rooms, nurses' stations, and consulting rooms to observe the work of medical staff and their interactions with patients. While in the hospital, I observed how boxes of chocolates and other food items circulated, and I heard patients in the corridors talk among themselves about envelopes in Lithuanian, Russian, and Polish. I conversed with doctors, nurses, patients, and their relatives about their experiences with the health-care system. I also conducted open-ended interviews with doctors of different generations, ranging from those in their first years of residency to those nearing retirement. I talked to patients, some of whom I interviewed in the hospital along with their relatives. I also spent time observing patients and their caregivers and socializing at their homes throughout Lithuania, in addition to attending birthday parties and other family celebrations. I found out that those who gave or did not cannot be divided into categories of poor/wealthy or low/middle/upper class. Within the same groups and even families, some gave while others did not, and they all still received the medical care they needed. There was no single logic of (not) giving.

Doctors and patients frequently asked me about my health-care experiences in the United States. They wanted to know how much I paid for health insurance and what I got in return, what the waiting times were, and how doctors communicated with their patients. They also inquired if envelopes existed in the United States, too, and whether patients complained about doctors and the health-care system. I told them about my own experiences and the debates about the state of health care. Oftentimes, after our conversations, patients nodded their heads and concluded that they did not have much to complain about, and doctors agreed that there were problems with health-care systems everywhere.

During the summers of 2012–14, winter of 2015, and spring of 2017, I returned to Lithuania and talked to patients, their relatives, and doctors. During follow-up visits I shared my findings with them. These conversations were invaluable for my writing process. An article based on the material from chapter two was translated into Lithuanian and published in 2018. Some of the interlocutors who appear in the book read that article and commented on it. Everyone, it seemed, wanted to understand how these envelopes worked and affected them. Sadly, two of my informants in the book—Jurgis and Brigita—have passed away.

I also traced the genealogy of health-care reform in postsocialist Lithuania to find out how informal payments became entangled with public health as a barrier to the emergence of business relations in the health-care sector. My archival research for this issue focused on the public discourse about informal monetary transactions in medicine to understand how these practices came to be seen as a problem and for whom. I studied the works of Lithuanian health-care policy scholars, documents of the Ministry of Health, and articles about health care in magazines and newspapers. During my stay in Lithuania, I also visited two private clinics. I interviewed the staff of TIL and officials of the Ministry of Health of Lithuania and the Prevention Department of the Special Economic Crimes Investigation. Finally, I drew on my own experience as a patient and a caregiver for family members as we navigated the health-care system in Lithuania and faced many of the same dilemmas that my future informants have.

I believe that social theory is a storytelling practice that allows us to narrate ambiguities and contradictions in discrete ways (Verran 2001). The life of the envelope begins not in the hospital or the outpatient clinic; it begins with storytelling and story. Beyond accounts of lived personal experience there are what I call the "canonical tales" of enveloped care. Stories about chocolate boxes and envelopes of money constitute a specific genre that contains elements of folk wisdom and folk tales while focusing on health-care encounters. These formulaic tales, which I have heard over many years, are different from the firsthand accounts that comprise this book's chapters. They dwell "in their own context of signs," as Kathleen Stewart (1996) observes, incorporating practices, fears, desires, hope, life changes, gratitude, and disappointment. Building on Roland Barthes's definition of myth as a form of speech chosen by history, a system of communication, and a concept filled with certain knowledge, I treat these tales as myth-like (Barthes 1972, 109–10, 122). I am less interested in their veracity, or in how fully they correspond to the reality of health care in Lithuania than I am in examining which elements change over time and with retelling, reflecting local histories and relations, and which remain the same. The tales enact relations and conceptualizations of the world that make realities possible. They do this by drawing maps of how to take care of people and things.

In other words, these stories are relations, and they make relations. Not only do they accompany and narrate the practice of caring, but they also constitute that practice (Certeau 1984). The canonical tales I heard were often accompanied by other stories, commentaries, and recollections of personal experiences. They also illustrate how enveloped encounters were not limited to health care but rather were a texture of life during Soviet socialism. They acted as a prologue to a conversation, an interlude, a transition, or a way of concluding an exchange, and I thread them between the chapters of this book in the same way. These tales weave the moral fabric of care and constitute a local epistemology of health and care.

Enveloped Lives

This book unpacks the relations that are bundled in the little white envelopes to detail how and why state officials, patients, doctors, and caretakers encounter, perceive, enact, and perpetuate this particular form of care. I begin by tracing health-care reform in Lithuania since the end of socialism in 1990. The first chapter, "From Bribes to Copayments," problematizes policies of transparency and the practices and ethics of payment in a market-based health-care system. Attempts to turn the money in envelopes into transparent copayments reveal how envelopes embody tensions over the informality, legality, or transparency of payments for health care. They also raise fundamental questions about values, shared responsibilities, inequality, and the cost of living in the postsocialist state. The chapter juxtaposes two different economies of health care: envelopes that resemble a human economy (in which money is social currency) and payments that are situated within a market economy.[16] Even though money is part of both economies of care, they are not the same. In the human economy of relationships, money is not necessarily a payment. In this chapter, I show how the calculative mechanism of envelopes and their valuation exceed the logic of the payment. Giving an envelope is a personal practice that is not based on market equivalences. It is meant to emphasize the distinctiveness of each person. This distinction can help us understand how the enveloped economy has resisted reform and continued to function for all these years.

Regardless of how people felt about the informal economy of giving, it seemed nearly impossible to escape the ubiquity and power of envelopes. Chapter 2, "Being Caught," focuses on the experiences of patients and their caregivers as they manage the network of relations, expectations, and desired outcomes wrapped up in enveloped care. Their stories illustrate how knowledge and beliefs about enveloped practices are transmitted, and how in that process envelopes have become imbued with both practical and symbolic efficacy. The envelope is both a mechanism for coping with the limitations of biomedicine in Lithuania and a healing force that, for some, can have a direct effect on the body. These dynamics lead to what I call "being caught" in the envelope. When they are "caught," patients and caregivers interpret all medical encounters through the lens of the envelope. A doctor's tone of voice or facial expression, the beckoning pockets of white coats, a nurse's suggestion "talk to the doctor," or slow computer systems all might be a sign of provocation. For some, that means being forced or pressured to deal with the ambiguous and anxiety-producing practice of figuring out how much and when to give. For others, it means feeling like if they do not participate, their health will suffer, either because of a disappointed doctor or because the envelope itself has healing powers. And those who do not give may still be indirectly roped into the system by family members who insist on giving. As the failure to eradicate the informal economy of envelopes illustrates, the health-care system itself is caught in the envelope.

If patients and their loved ones are caught in the ambiguities of the system, doctors are too in their roles as both medical providers and caregivers for their own ailing families. Chapter 3, "I Am a Doctor," describes how doctors deal with enveloped practices. Because offering money and gifts to medical providers is so engrained in the Lithuanian health care system, becoming a good doctor involves learning not only to be competent and caring but how to navigate encounters with envelopes. Young doctors doing their residency in hospitals must develop a personal ethical code for dealing with envelopes. On accepting one for the first time, some doctors experience a sense of failure or betrayal of professional ideals. With time, they come to define their ethical position and justify accepting envelopes as long as they are not asking for them. This is both a way of interacting with patients and defining the boundaries of acceptable practice and doctor-patient relations. I discuss how doctors distinguish between payments, bribes, and gifts; between good and unscrupulous doctors; and how they perceive challenges to medical authority and the commodification of care. This chapter also illustrates the shifting economies of health from the medical provider's perspective. It recounts how doctors perceive their working conditions and the new constraints they have encountered in the postsocialist state. These realities affect their own opinions on the practice of envelopes in the context of ongoing health-care reform.

The last chapter, "Collective Care: Relations of Obligation," is a reflection on enveloped care as particularly bittersweet. Through the story of a small-town baker and his family, dating back to 1944, I underscore how offerings of food and money have connected families, neighbors, and doctors in what I call "caring collectives." These assemblages are activated by the will to care for the sick within existing conditions. They are a vital element of enveloped care that puts the emphasis not on a patient's autonomy but on interdependency and kinship. In the process, they knit together medical practitioners and patients with all their relations. These relationships—mediated by money, food, or other objects—sustained lives during wars, occupations, and economic transformations and created a particular economy of health that now poses challenges to neoliberal health care reforms. Health care reform projects that seek more efficiency and transparency do not necessarily deliver better care. However bittersweet enveloped care is, it expresses the desire for affordable, sensible, and personalized care that has space for gratitude.

The envelope is a polyvalent object and a concept that resists simple explanations based on rationality, socioeconomic status, institutional violence, corruption, generosity, or the force of habit. The envelope is an interpretative framework through which patients and caregivers make sense of medical encounters and relationships. Moreover, the envelope is part of the treatment and healing process itself. It expresses a situated relationship to caring, one that leads to more nuanced understandings of good and bad care. It is an embodiment of the uncertainty and ambiguity people continue to experience in the context of institutionalized medicine in both capitalist and socialist regimes.

Interlude I

THE CIRCULATING CHOCOLATE BOX

Once, a friend of a friend had to see a doctor . . . so he went to see the family doctor and gave him a box of chocolates. You know, you have to give something to the doctors. The box was marked. A note for the doctor was left inside the box. The doctor took the box and put it on the shelf in his office. The man received the help he was expecting and forgot about the box, until one day, he himself received a box of chocolates from a neighbor who needed a favor. The box looked similar to the one he had given to the family doctor; then again, all boxes of chocolates looked similar because under socialism there were only a few varieties available. The only distinctive feature was a ribbon around the box, which also looked familiar. When the man opened the box of chocolates, he found the note that he had written for the doctor. The sell-by date on the box was two weeks earlier. It was the same box he had given to the doctor.

Pranas, a sixty-seven-year-old retired engineer, told me this story in the fall of 2010. Sitting with him in his living room in the city of Klaipeda were his wife Janina, their daughter Rita, and their granddaughter Barbora. All of them laughed when Pranas finished the story.

When I spoke about my project researching envelopes, whether in Lithuania or my current home in California talking to Lithuanians living here, people often responded: "I can tell you a story that happened to a friend of a friend. It is a story about a box of chocolates. It's a true story." I could usually guess what was coming. Details of the story such as the time period, the occupation of the patient, the doctor's specialization, the location, and the list of people who successively receive the box may change, yet the central elements are consistent: a patient gives a box of chocolates to a doctor; the doctor and successive recipients regift the unopened box until it eventually returns to the original patient.[1]

I have heard this tale from a wide range of people, including my parents, in-laws, engineers, artists, clerks, teachers, a farmer, and a young art critic whom I had just met. Whether it is set in the socialist era or contemporary Lithuania, it is always told as having happened to a friend of a friend. The protagonists include not only the patient and the doctor but the box of chocolates itself.

"Grandpa, how did the box get back to your friend? I didn't get that," asked six-year-old Barbora. Then, Pranas, the storyteller, retraced the journey of the box of chocolates. "The friend of a friend was a driving instructor; so he gave the box to the doctor; the doctor gave the box to a mechanic who looked after his car; the mechanic's wife gave the box to a kindergarten teacher; the kindergarten teacher gave the box to a saleswoman; and the saleswoman gave the box to her driving instructor, who was the patient in the first instance."

In other versions of the story that referred to the socialist period, the people who passed the box of chocolates around to facilitate a transaction or as a thank-you gift included a pharmacist, a nurse, a tailor, a hairdresser, a theater box-office clerk, a teacher, a bureaucrat, an accountant, an engineer, a tax inspector, a secretary, and a sales associate. In versions of the tale set after the 1990s, people no longer gave chocolates to salespeople or mechanics, but the story began to feature a new figure, the tax inspector. This shift reflects the fact that there was no longer a shortage of material goods, and service industries were becoming privatized. Yet the story always begins with and includes a doctor. Although late socialism might have been defined by shortages of many things, including medications and medical technologies, there was no shortage of doctors. Moreover, almost everyone has to deal with doctors, not only for the treatment of illness but also for check-ups required for admission to a preschool or university, getting or renewing a driver's license, and certain occupations.

The brand of chocolates mentioned in the story also changed, reflecting increased consumer choice after the Soviet era. (In the mid-1990s, one brand of locally produced chocolates was advertised on TV as "the best bribe.") In stories dating from the Soviet period, one frequently mentioned brand was Assorti, a large box of assorted chocolates that was considered luxurious. Others included Paukščių Pienas (a medium-sized box of chocolate-covered marshmallows), Sostinė (chocolates with brandy), Mon Cheri, and Laima. When the tale referred to brands of chocolates made in independent Lithuania, the cast of characters included an accountant, a tax inspector, friends, other doctors, and state officials. Sometimes storytellers did not name the brand.

The distinguishing mark of the box, which enabled the original giver to identify it when it returned, varied. Sometimes the box was marked by a colored ribbon (red, pink, blue, gold), an expiration date, a small pen or pencil marking (a dot or a letter), or a slightly bent corner. Different versions of the tale describe the journey of the box of chocolates through the capital city, Vilnius, as well as other cities such as Kaunas and Klaipeda. Even if the patient lived in a village, the box traveled to the city. If it contained money, the amount might be stipulated in rubles or litai; the box might contain only chocolates or include a thank-you card or note. The doctor who received it might be an eye doctor, surgeon, cardiologist, family doctor, psychiatrist, or gynecologist.

As long as it remained unopened, the box retained its ability to contribute to healing patients, fixing cars, making teachers and students happier, or obtaining fabrics, meat, books, theater tickets, the right size or model of shoes, or valuable information. The box stopped circulating once it was recognized by the original giver, or perhaps because its expiration date had passed; otherwise, it could theoretically circulate indefinitely. Its journey inscribes a circle of people who otherwise do not know each other personally.

The transmission of the box echoes the Kula ring, the process of ceremonial exchange described by Bronislaw Malinowski. Bracelets and necklaces circulate in different directions but never leave the social circle, around which is a "network of relationships, and . . . naturally the whole forms one interwoven fabric" (Malinowski [1922] 2010, 92). As in the Kula ring, the boxes and relationships bind people who are not otherwise close, although the relationships are not necessarily enduring ones. In contrast to the items circulated in the Kula ring, the box usually is not displayed in public but hidden in a closet or drawer or on a shelf. The box, unlike the decorative objects of the Kula ring, also has a practical use, and this very quality might prevent the completion of its journey. Yet its circulation illustrates the interconnectedness of multiple people otherwise not directly connected. Gifts and reciprocal favors form affectively charged relationships (Yang 1994, 171).

This tale could also be seen as a classic illustration of *blat*, the system of informal contacts, connections, favors, and exchanges, mediated by rhetoric of friendship that flourished in the Soviet era. *Blat* was a matter of belonging to a circle of acquaintances. According to Alena Ledeneva, the system arose from the structural characteristics of Soviet socialism: "the particular combination of shortages and, even if repressed, consumerism; from a paradox between an ideology of equality and the practice of differentiation through privileges and closed distribution systems" (1998, 36, 40). *Blat* acted as a mechanism that made the state-controlled economy somewhat workable (Humphrey 2002, 138). A box of chocolates that traversed multiple encounters and relations would belong to a category that Ledeneva calls "blat-gifts," which she characterizes as "redundant transactions used for the construction of small social worlds" (1998, 153). In the canonical tales, the traveling box accompanies and facilitates relations among a variety of people, creating, sustaining, and expanding social worlds.

Although the giver's original marking or decoration of the box—the characteristic that allows it to be identified later—can perhaps be seen as a personal touch, it is not too personal to preclude regifting the box to another person. Gifts such as boxes of chocolates and bottles of brandy, according to Jennifer Patico, "like the relationships they objectify, strike a balance between personalization and anonymity"; that is, they fall between kin-like relations and market transactions (2002, 357). The box of chocolates is both a relation between people and a moral aesthetics of action (Humphrey 2012, 23).

"Oh, you are interested in boxes, bottles, and things like that? I could be your subject! I gave a box of chocolates to the doctor when my mother was in the hospital. Funny things happen with these boxes. . . . I have a story to tell you," said a young art critic in skinny jeans and fashionable cardigan, who just minutes earlier had been updating me on what I should see while visiting London's Tate Modern. "Once a friend of a friend had to see a doctor . . ."

FROM BRIBES TO COPAYMENTS
Transforming Health Care in Lithuania

In 2004, Transparency International Lithuania (TIL) created a public service video, *Don't Bribe: A Bribe Is Not a Guarantee,* which criticized alleged bribery in the medical profession. It aimed to educate patients while also promoting a new culture of transparency. Since its establishment in 2000, TIL has become a vocal actor in fighting alleged corruption in the Lithuanian health-care system. Along with a neoliberal think-tank, the Free Market Institute, TIL has advocated for transforming informal payments between patients and their doctors into legal and transparent copayments. The video appeared on national TV and was shown in TIL-sponsored seminars to doctors, journalists, and activists to mark the beginning of new standards, ethics, and a culture of transparency. The discourse of transparency encapsulated a particular historical moment in Lithuania: a departure from its Soviet past and its entry into the European Union (EU).

The video shows an operating room in a modern hospital. The medical team is waiting for their patient to be rolled in for surgery. Once the patient arrives, and the doctor is at his bedside, we see a second patient being rolled in. This second patient lifts his head, examines the room, and puts 200 litai into the surgeon's pocket. The camera zooms in on this transaction and freezes.

After the doctor takes the money, the first patient (supposedly without money) is moved off the operating table, and the patient with money is moved into his place. The camera zooms in again on the banknote. This vignette is followed by the message on the screen: "A bribe is not a guarantee. There will always be someone who will pay more" (*Kyšis ne garantas. Atsiras kas duos daugiau*). Then the action resumes. A third patient is rolled into the operating room, this time

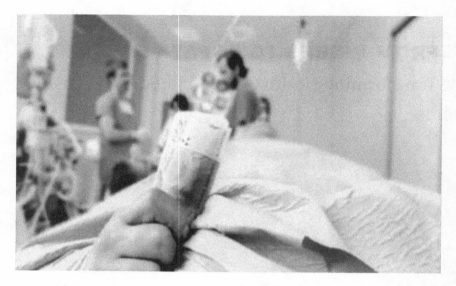

FIGURE 1 Patient holds money while being rolled into the operating room. Screen capture. Source: PSA, *Don't Bribe*, Transparency International Lithuania, 2004, www.transparency.lt.

with a briefcase full of money, like a scene in a mafia film. This time the viewer does not see the patient's face, only the open briefcase full of cash. The video ends with the message: "Don't give" (*Neduok*) and the information that it was sponsored by the EU.

The image of the second patient holding money in his hand (figure 1) became a signature illustration for anticorruption campaigns and appeared in Transparency International's *Global Corruption Report 2006*.[1] TIL experts, along with experts from the Free Market Institute, recommended legalizing informal payments by turning them into formal copayments. This transformation from one operational logic to another and the reactions to it from doctors and the general public underscore the tensions that have arisen with the attempts to rationalize health care in postsocialist, capitalist Lithuania.

The TIL argues that the current practice of informal payments in the health-care system is not viable. As Darius, an activist with the organization, explained to me, the goal of the video was to show that Lithuanian patients are forced into competitive bidding for the attention of doctors because of a lack of transparency and a self-reinforcing belief in the efficacy of those bribes. In a similar vein, the health economist Janos Kornai explains, "Gratuities cause confusion among patients. The market is not transparent and the prices are unclear. Everyone is hesitant about giving too much or too little. Patients vie with each other, which

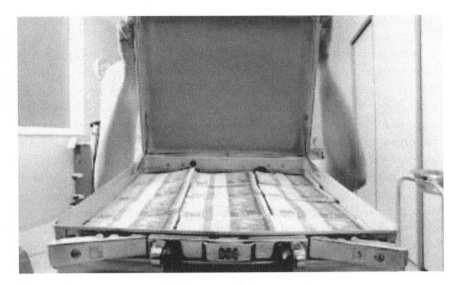

FIGURE 2   Patient holds a briefcase full of money. Screen capture.
Source: PSA, *Don't Bribe*, Transparency International Lithuania, 2004,
www.transparency.lt.

pushes up the prevailing rates of gratuity" (Kornai, 2000: 172). Current health-
care reform documents also use the words "nontransparent income/payments"
and "illegal copayments" synonymously.[2]

The concepts of transparency and rationality date back to the Enlightenment
and are intrinsic to the notion of modernity. They are often contrasted with the
climate of doubt, irrationality, and tradition that purportedly preceded it (Sanders
and West 2003). According to this modern logic, the lack of transparency in
transactions and relations between doctors and patients makes patients compete
for doctors' attention and pushes up the cost of care. However, processes and
relations between doctors and patients, including giving envelopes, are not subject to the logic of competition prevalent in a market economy. Patients and their
caregivers are not competing with others in the amounts of money they give to
doctors and nurses. Quite the opposite, they were careful not to give too much.

In summing up the effectiveness of TIL's various actions—the video, posters
in cities and on public transportation, hotlines, and even public performances
in which people dressed up as envelopes and circulated a petition written from
their perspective—Darius acknowledged that these don't give campaigns are not
working. It is not enough to deter doctors from accepting envelopes, he noted,
"because people may worry about why what they were giving wasn't accepted."
Despite the purportedly corrupting effect of the envelopes, the health-care

system continues to function, while the transparency campaigns, as the activist metaphorically put it, were approaching a dead end.

When we talked in 2010 about TIL's attempts to increase transparency in Lithuania, Darius expressed his frustration: "The levels of bribery in the health-care system haven't changed in the last ten years. People still see a bribe as an effective way to solve their problems. They are prepared to bribe. We are trying to prove that corruption is bad and transparency is good; it is that simple." The organization had been tracking the levels of corruption through an annual survey of the perception of corruption and illustrating it graphically on a "corruption map." According to a 2011 map, 60 percent of patients gave envelopes with money to their doctors.[3] Twelve percent of those patients said that they were "provoked" by doctors to do so, and the remaining 88 percent said it was their decision to thank the doctor.[4] Another study, conducted by the Association of Private Health Care Organizations in 2016, states that roughly half of the patients who thanked their doctors "felt a moral obligation" or did so because they thought doctors' salaries were inadequate.[5] The surveys consistently showed that approximately 50 percent of respondents engaged in health-care-related "bribing practices."[6]

According to Darius, TIL was frustrated that doctors saw no problems with informal payments. The doctors' union had not been cooperative; indeed, the organization opposes defining any monetary transactions between patients and doctors as bribes.[7] Although the union condemns extorting, provoking, and accepting money before surgeries, it considers money, food, or other items that patients freely give to be gifts and expressions of thanks. The representatives of the doctors' union publicly supported the inclusion of the Medical Gift Law in the Civil Code in 2000 that aimed to legalize gifts to the doctors.

"We had high hopes in 2004, when Lithuania was granted EU membership," Darius sighed nostalgically. The organization created numerous educational campaigns to change the minds of Lithuanian patients and doctors so that they would not, in Darius's words, "become socialized within this culture of bribery and corruption, but slowly start changing." For him, it was disheartening that Lithuania was not "truly Western." Even if the envelopes were part of a cultural tradition, Darius argued, "they have to be transparent, cultural but transparent."

In 2010, I showed *Don't Bribe* to a group of preschool teachers and staff (eleven women and one man) in the city of Klaipėda and asked them to share their thoughts.[8] They laughed as they watched the video: "Look, look! The full briefcase." They nodded their heads and agreed, "Oh, yes, we give money," but they were not necessarily happy about doing so. Very quickly, the viewers turned to their own stories of envelopes and medical encounters. They talked about anxieties, illness, provocations, caring and uncaring doctors, extortion, and grati-tude. They corrected each other, adding more layers to every narrative. It was obvious that the group had shared stories of their health-care experiences quite a few times. "I always ask you about the amount," said a music teacher to a senior colleague. "And I ask you," she continued pointing to an accountant, "and you," looking at the janitor, "because you get sick more often." Everybody was asking questions of everybody else. People of similar income levels were sharing their stories and using them as references for how much to give.

One of the teachers remarked, referring to the video, "One day, medicine might become so expensive that you will need to pay for everything—every visit, everything. You might need that briefcase." The group perceived the huge differ-ence in payments between the patients portrayed in the video not as a current reality but as a future possibility. What this group of Lithuanians, of modest income, wanted was caring, unlimited, free, and universal health care. Envelopes were not the biggest problem of health care for them. It was the price of pharma-ceuticals that posed the heaviest financial burden for the patients.[9]

This chapter explores tensions in the changing political economy of health that are embodied in enveloped practices. The tensions over informality and transparency of payments for health care epitomize the contestation of values that foreground health and care in postsocialist capitalism. How did questions of copayments, envelopes, and privatization become entangled in Lithuania? How did informal payments become coupled with the need to privatize health care? In this chapter I address these questions from three angles. I begin with the history of Lithuanian health care under socialism through tales about Lenin and Stalin and their involvement with the practice of giving envelopes. I then examine the twenty-year history of health-care reform projects focusing on changes in public hospitals. Finally, I look at the relation between the development of private health care and the drive to eliminate informal payments.

Understanding the tensions between different interpretations of enveloped practices in health care, whether as a cultural issue, an economic problem, or a matter of transparency and corruption, is indispensable for grappling with the present-day Lithuanian definition of health and its policies and practices. Doctors' salaries, envelopes with money that patients give to doctors (whether conceptualized as gifts, bribes, informal payments, or nontransparent income), and the future of public health are linked tightly in debates regarding the past, present, and the future of health care in Lithuania. These tensions, rooted in the history of socialist and postsocialist transformations, provide sociopolitical context for understanding the persistence of enveloped care and how it is driven by the will to care.

The Breakup: Postsocialist Capitalist Transformations

On March 11, 1990, after fifty years of Soviet occupation, Lithuania regained its independence, the first of the Soviet republics to do so. On the same day, it reinstated the 1938 constitution of the Lithuanian Republic and reestablished the right to own private property. The new state immediately began the process of undoing the totalitarian Soviet regime, along with its state socialism. Lithuanian intellectuals were inspired by advocates of classic liberalism like Friedrich Hayek's *The Road to Serfdom* (Hajekas 1991), that was highly critical of centrally planned economies and believed that the intrinsic organizing principles of governance should be the freedom of the individual and the market. The state embarked on a project of conversion from a planned economy and a police state to deregulation and personal freedoms, from overregulation to deregulation, from compulsory work to freedom of choice in employment.

In this period of massive change, health care was an arena in which there was continuity. Informal payments for health care persevered alongside new neoliberal arrangements, such as efficiency, competition, and management of hospitals as enterprises. This is perhaps not surprising. Alexei Yurchak (2002, 2003) shows how the "entrepreneurial governmentality" within Soviet state socialism—the coexistence of personalized and official business/economic arrangements—fluidly merged into neoliberal arrangements aimed at transforming the "apparatchiks" into capitalists. Johanna Bockman (2011) also demonstrates the linkages between Eastern European socialism and neoliberalism. Michel Foucault's analysis of postwar German socialism and neoliberalism in his lectures on biopolitics at the College de France (2008) is also useful for thinking through the relation between state socialism and neoliberalism in the former Soviet bloc. In Lithuania, as in postwar Germany, the totalitarian regime's atrocities against the people, and those of its collaborators within the regime, were denounced publicly and in court trials. The first steps of the newly elected Lithuanian government were to outlaw the Communist Party and Soviet symbols and to initiate a market economy. These processes often referenced and followed the logic of de-Nazification. The architects of market reform in Lithuania, such as Prime Minister Kazimiera Prunskiene, a professor of economics, also referenced Germany's "social market" as a model for Lithuania, and so did Lithuanian social policy experts (Aidukaite, Bogdanova, and Guogis 2012, 339).[10] Lithuanian reforms were thus inspired by the application of the ideas of the German ordoliberals, which Foucault invokes to explore the notions of biopolitics, the market, and neoliberalism.

Foucault asserts that socialism has a distinct historical, economic, and administrative rationality but "no governmental rationality" (2008, 92). Socialism worked, according to him, through its connection to liberal governmentality and the governmentality of the police state, functioning as "the internal logic of an administrative apparatus," with perhaps other forms of governmentality, too (Foucault 2008, 92). If we take up Foucault's proposal that socialism is not an alternative to liberalism, and instead examine its technologies of governing, then the transition from socialism to capitalism is not so much a switch to the easily spread "free market," but rather a set of reconfigurations with their own accelerations, blockages, and arrangements (Collier 2012). Drawing on Foucault, rationalization within governance can be viewed as an attempt to maximize the effects of governing while reducing costs. In this sense, the rationalization of health care involves not only marketization but also the reduction of its political and economic costs (Foucault 2008, 318) by governing people's conduct—that is, by interpreting individual behavior, social relations, and governmental practices through the analytics of market forces. In this case, the market is not a fixed notion but always contingent, and biopolitics and markets are mutually constituted.[11]

Lithuania's breakup from the Soviet Union coincided with the rise of neoliberal governmentality in the United States, Latin America, and Europe. In the late 1980s and 1990s, tenets of deregulation and privatization—such as the creation of internal markets, ideas of entrepreneurship, and competition—were being introduced to socialized health-care systems in Western European countries (Day 2016; Oliver 2012; Waldby and Cooper 2008). The push in Eastern European nations for operational and economic efficiency in health care, to be attained through the logic of the market, was in tune with these changes elsewhere (Mollaghan and Dao 2016). In 1993–94, the large-scale privatization of Lithuanian state-owned factories, apartments, and services began. "Market reform" was the official agenda, supported by the International Monetary Fund and the European Union.

Despite these changes, most Eastern European countries have kept access to free health care (Kornai 2001, 143). Instead of eradicating all forms of Soviet social welfare, the reforms selectively reconfigured social norms and inherited material structures (Collier 2011, 3). In 2001, Kornai described the health-care situation as "a fragment of socialism [that] had survived in the midst of a capitalist market economy" (2001, 5). According to Kornai, the slow pace of privatization in health care may have been due in large part to practices of informal payments: "The prevalence and demoralizing effect of gratuities are one of the main brakes on the emergence of straightforward private activity and respectable business relations in the health sector" (2001, 175). Indeed, if society aspires to a privatized and reconfigured health-care system, envelopes could be seen as an impediment. If we question whether privatized health care could really improve the lives of people, increase affordability, and reduce inequalities, then it is far from clear that the envelopes have a demoralizing effect on the health-care system by preserving the existing order.

Thank Lenin and Stalin; Or, Doctors Do Not Need Salaries

"Good doctors are never poor." Patients and their caregivers repeated this aphorism often when they commented on doctors' low salaries. The point was that even if doctors were underpaid, grateful patients would always adequately compensate the good ones.

This belief has a long history. "Patients always gave money and food to their doctors. That is why Stalin wanted to eliminate salaries for doctors, so that they would collect (*susirinkti*) payment from the patients, like priests," I was told in 2008 by an official of the Patients' Fund, who worked for many years drafting and implementing elements of the ongoing health-care reform in Lithuania. This official had practiced as a doctor in one of the regional towns before becoming a politician and then a health-care bureaucrat. For him, the presence of envelopes in doctor-patient encounters was an unsolvable problem if even Stalin, notorious for his tight control, acknowledged it. He sounded nostalgic. Perhaps he was even a Stalin sympathizer. I wrote his story in my journal but later forgot about it, only to be reminded of it when I heard a similar story later.

Comparing doctors to priests—whose parishioners support them materially while submitting to their moral authority—casts the patient-doctor relationship as an example of the self-organized play in relationships of power. Informal payments to doctors fall within the realm of alms or tips that, in turn, differentiate good and bad doctors. Stalin's supposed inability to prevent doctors from taking money is an argument for turning a blind eye to this practice in Lithuania today. Attempts to inscribe informal payments as gifts in the Civil Code of Lithuania, the opinions expressed by representatives of the Lithuanian Doctors' Union, and local scholars of health-care policy reflect this line of thought.

Four years later, in 2012, Laimutis Paškevičius, the president of the Association of Private Health Care Organizations, told a similar story while expressing his disappointment with the slow pace of health-care privatization. His version, however, invoked Lenin. Newspapers and internet portals repeated the tale, quoting the president as saying: "The system is deep-rooted. If we look closely at the Soviet era, it is said that when Lenin was deciding on salaries, he said that doctors would get money from their patients. Perhaps that's why their salaries are low."[12]

The official used this version of the tale to condemn the practice of envelopes and to suggest that the way to finally end informal payments and solve the problem of low salaries was through privatizing health care.

This second story reflects a different sort of problematization. Lenin's paying doctors low salaries is represented as a faulty decision, one that affected the whole socialist system. In this version of the tale, free public health care is held responsible for several evils: underpaid doctors, patients' lack of responsibility for their own health, and the existence of informal payments. This story resonated with the arguments and interpretations made by free-market advocates and private health-care institutions; the only way to eliminate these problems is to introduce a system of official medical copayments, while opening the health sector to private capital and the real market.

These two versions of the story reflect the tension and ambiguity of health-care reform initiatives and the current health-care system, which works through enveloped practices and resists significant shifts to it. They illustrate the complex relationship between the state, doctors, patients, and enveloped medicine with references to faith, economy, and history. They also represent a kind of origin myth for enveloped practices, asserting the role of Lenin and Stalin in creating and enabling the system of envelopes. These stories also challenge the official socialist position that all doctors were equal (good and bad doctors all received the same salary). Both stories compare doctors to priests, whose practices of religious rites and pastoral care are financially supported by donations from parishioners. Even though the Soviet state highly restricted and regulated priests' lives during socialism, doctors' lives supposedly escaped such regulations. In that sense, it confirms the exclusivity of the medical profession, subtly suggesting that biomedicine (and science) replaced religion in the Soviet Union.

Maryna Bazylevych documents another version of this story in her ethnography of Ukrainian physicians. She alleges that Lenin rejected the idea of doctors' salaries, saying, "Good physicians will always be able to feed themselves and their families, and bad physicians—well, we do not need them!" (2009, 77). The Ukrainian doctors used the story to illustrate the double standard of Soviet morality, when "earning unofficial income was deemed wrong, but on the other hand, physicians were still expected to earn additional income" (Bazylevych 2009, 77). It seems that doctors in the Ukrainian version wanted appropriate state regulation, even while seriously doubting the very possibility of it. During my conversations with Lithuanian doctors, however, the stories about Lenin and Stalin did not come up. This may indicate differing local standards of ethics and morality, as well as a certain level of comfort with the practice of envelopes and a desire not for more intervention and oversight by the state but for its partial disengagement.

As I noted in the introduction, the history of informal payments to doctors in Eastern Europe may predate the Soviet regime and the associated economies of shortage. Following state-modernization initiatives in nineteenth-century imperial Russia, doctors were treated as salaried workers (Bazylevych 2009, 27; Keshavjee 2014; Knauss 1980). Doctors, who were from the lower strata of society, received a basic salary and could charge fees to patients on a sliding scale, with the poorest patients paying nothing. Thus, payments for health care were predicated largely on doctor-patient relationships. Beginning in 1940, with the Soviet occupation of Lithuania, the state-run health-care system, in which all treatment was officially free, struggled to eradicate monetary relations between patients and doctors. Most of the patients ignored exhortations to end the bourgeois habit of giving money to doctors (Vaiseta 2015, 54–55).

In the middle of the nineteenth century, when Lithuania was part of the Russian empire, the state offered stipends for the children of serfs and peasants to study medicine. Later, these peasant children became the leaders of the cultural revival movement and the modern Lithuanian nation. Doctors (along with priests) organized and distributed underground newspapers in the then-forbidden Lithuanian language, fought for workers' rights, organized public health campaigns, and wrote the texts of the national anthem and the declaration of independence in 1918. They were advocates of social democracy and universal health care during the interwar period as well. After the Soviet occupation, many doctors left Lithuania and became refugees, while others were deported to labor camps in Siberia. In the late 1980s and 1990s, doctors were active in the independence movement.

Local histories, and the tales of Lenin and Stalin, convey how the socialist state project singled out doctors, allowing them to continue prerevolutionary payment practices that sustained them during this period as well. This made the medical care/health system an exceptional configuration in the Soviet state assemblage, constituted by prerevolutionary and socialist elements, while combining both a strong state presence (the right to health, the development of health-care infrastructure) and the allowable exceptionality of doctor-patient transactions. Enveloped practices repeatedly escaped regulation by the socialist state's biopolitics; doctors' and patients' relationships were left to partial self-governance. Sean Brotherton (2012) observes similar manifestations of self-governance linked to the health-care sector in post-Soviet Cuba. The proliferation of spaces of informality illustrates how individual practices of care that contradict the socialist state can both escape and maintain it at the same time. Brotherton (2012, 184) argues that it is "a unique form of biopolitical self-governance," a process that was not entirely unrelated or incomparable to the construction of the Western autonomous subject.

With the end of the socialist state and the rise of capitalist markets in Lithuania, this form of self-governance, with its entitlements, expectations, and relations, has not become completely commodified. It continues to circumvent the regulations of both the state and the market. Enveloped care thus represents a distinct biopolitical form that continues to develop and may even offer new configurations of health care and remuneration.

Coupling Bribes and Privatization

The reconfiguration of the health-care system has been a long and bumpy process. Lithuania, like other post-Soviet countries, inherited a chronically underfunded health-care system. The Soviet Union spent only 3 percent of GDP on health care in 1989. Its health-care system lagged in technological development, life expectancy, and other health indicators (Gudžinskas 2012, 64, 65).[13] In the first decade after the fall of the USSR, the Baltic states were the only ones that reformed their health-care systems. The Lithuanian Ministry of Health attempted the gradual optimization and rationalization of health care through decentralization and partial privatization. Health-care reform proposals drafted in 1990, immediately after the country became independent from the Soviet Union, included plans to end informal payments. One of the first studies of the reform proposals noted: "The health-care system, inherited from the Soviet past, even with the surpluses of doctors, creates an artificial shortage of services which allows the system of bribes to exist" (Černiauskas 1996, 30). Thus, it was officially acknowledged that the new state had to deal with the legacy of the Soviet political economy.

Between the 1990s and 2012, there were three planned stages of health reform, based on advice received from the World Bank and from German, Scandinavian, and local experts (mostly affiliated with the Free Market Institute).[14] Many of these experts recommended reducing the number of facilities and doctors to increase efficiency and reduce costs. Despite this advice Lithuania retained a dense network of polyclinics and hospitals. This inherited, solid network of health-care institutions became a tense reform issue in regard to the maintenance of the population's health, keeping state-funded jobs, and increasing efficiency. The country has more practicing doctors and hospital beds than the EU average.[15] Hospital stays are also longer than the EU average, even though these numbers have been slowly declining (Merkšiūnaitė 2017; Starkiene 2012).[16]

In discussions in the early 1990s, the health-care reform group was split over whether to allow private companies and voluntary, supplemental health insurance into the health-care system (Černiauskas 1996, 32). There was a clash between radicals (mostly represented by young doctors) and moderates. The former advocated for the rapid privatization of health-care institutions and for citizens' ability to freely choose an insurance company, while the latter fought to keep existing health-care institutions and their benefits for the majority, even though they agreed to partial privatization (for pharmaceuticals and dentistry) (Jankauskienė 2000, 33). In 1995, the group decided to adopt a publicly financed health-care model.

In the first stage of reform, health-care funding was disconnected from the state budget. In 1996, Seimas, the Lithuanian parliament, passed legislation creating two institutional bodies—the National Health Insurance Fund (Valstybinė Ligonių Kasa) and the National Health Insurance Council—to ensure and regulate public health-care financing separately from the state budget. Health care was funded primarily by payroll taxes and supplemented by public funding to account for unemployed people. The National Health Insurance Fund reimbursed hospitals and outpatient clinics for treating patients rather than providing direct funding from state or municipal budgets. These changes ushered in a system of quotas and limits on care: waiting times for treatment grew longer, and hospital stays grew shorter. Under the reforms, long waits for treatment have become a major complaint about public health care.

Another major shift was the institution of the primary-care doctor as the gatekeeper to specialized consultations. During socialism, patients had been free to consult any doctor associated with the outpatient clinics serving their residential area, based partially on self-diagnosis (Skultans 2007). The reform required patients to obtain a referral from the family doctor to see a specialist. In theory, this change increased patient choice because patients were no longer limited to consulting the doctors at the nearest polyclinic. In practice, most patients remained bound to the local polyclinics because they were closest to their homes. Most patients and doctors described this change as an inconvenience. "Patients come and ask for referrals to the doctors they already know. I issue them referrals. Sometimes it is nonsense, when someone with a broken foot has to see me before a trauma specialist in our polyclinic," commented Rita, a family doctor in a large polyclinic in Vilnius. A prominent cardiologist commented, "I don't like much of what has been done. The system of family doctors is not functioning well. I think that the Soviet system, when everyone could decide which doctors to see, was better for the patient. What is a family doctor now—a gatekeeper, a dispatcher (*dispečeris*), sending patients to the specialists? The older system wasn't bad, but it was badly funded."

Doctors often emphasized a disconnect between primary care doctors and tertiary care facilities (university and regional hospitals). Some argued that family doctors with insufficient qualifications evaded responsibility by referring patients to specialists unnecessarily. Family doctors complained about the increased number of patients and waiting times. Doctors were unanimous that it used to be easier for patients to see a specialist. One emergency room doctor told me, "There will not be enough financing, ever. I don't think this rationalization and centralization of hospitals will save money. Everybody is glued to their chairs; clan mentality and bureaucracy will still flourish. I agree that there are too many hospitals but not enough care institutions." In other words, changes intended to increase efficiency did not necessarily translate into more or better care, shorter lines, happier doctors and patients, or even more efficiency. Most of the doctors described the reform as one long, never-ending process. No one talked about the stages of the reform that were inscribed in the health-care reform projects and documents. Every four years, after each parliamentary election, there was enthusiasm for speeding up the privatization and rationalization of the health-care system or rescinding the changes that had been made before.

Despite the large network of hospitals and polyclinics, in the 1990s many facilities were poorly equipped and lacked basic supplies. In 2000, the state borrowed 84 million litai from the World Bank to modernize health-care infrastructure (update diagnostic technologies, operating rooms, hospital buildings, and so on). At the time, experts blamed the lack of medical equipment and technological backwardness on the practice of informal payments. If these were transformed into copayments, according to this logic, the hospitals would have enough money to pay doctors more and improve their facilities. A few private diagnostic centers were portrayed widely in the media as an example of technological advancement and excellent consumer service. This logic fits neatly with the introduction of official voluntary copayments for elective procedures and premium service. Thus, private health care was presented as the only feasible alternative to the troubled public health-care system.

In 1994–95, Lithuania had fewer than one hundred hospital beds in private medical facilities, and 90 percent of doctors worked at state hospitals and polyclinics.[17] In the late 1990s, private polyclinics, maternity clinics, and diagnostic centers were established. Initially, most of their patients were foreigners living in Lithuania. Few Lithuanians used the private clinics because, as the director of one of the first clinics explained to me, they were "not used to private medicine and to paying for it. We have to teach people not to pay bribes but to go to private institutions, where it is very clear what people are paying for." What looked straightforward to the director was not clear at all to the patients like Lucija, who were not sure how their money would be used, or how they would impact doctors' lives and patient care.

Many attempts to establish a fully functioning private hospital failed. A revealing example is the private Heart Surgery Clinic (Širdies Chirurgijos Centras), a joint venture with the Japanese Marubeni Corporation, which in 1995, with a guarantee from the state, invested 58.9 million litai to open a private facility in Vilnius. The clinic went bankrupt in 2003, largely because it could not attract Lithuanian patients. It was sold for only 10 million litai to a retailer of building materials, Senukai.[18] Another scheme to privatize two polyclinics in Vilnius also failed in 2006. Advised by the Free Market Institute, the municipality of Vilnius came up with a plan to privatize two primary health-care units. The mayor, Arturas Zuokas, a proponent of neoliberal politics, argued that health care needed to be privatized because the Lithuanian health-care system rated poorly by EU standards.[19] In 2005, Vilnius citizens blocked an intersection near Naujoji Vilnia polyclinic, protesting the possible privatization of the outpatient clinic. The following year, Lithuanian Unions' Confederation organized protests against plans to privatize polyclinics.[20] Eventually, these protests from unions, doctors, and patients put this privatization plan on hold.

Until the 2010s, the gap between private and public health-care institutions and diagnostic centers was not only aesthetic. Private health-care institutions, while offering comforts that were often missing in poorly equipped, run-down buildings, still lacked enough patients. Between 2007 and 2013, the Lithuanian health-care system received 238.349 million euros for infrastructure upgrades.[21] In 2009–10, I revisited hospitals and polyclinics that I had been to as a patient and caregiver years earlier. After reading academic and local media discussions on the decaying state of health care in Eastern Europe, I had low expectations. To my surprise, except for the emergency room in the hospital where I did part of my fieldwork, most places seemed very orderly, clean, and up to date. Public polyclinics and hospitals in major cities occupied spacious buildings with specialized care units, where hundreds of full-time doctors and nurses served thousands of patients. The public health-care institutions lacked the sleek, modernist design and hotel-like atmosphere of a private clinic I visited in the outskirts of Vilnius, but they were modest and clean. The staff was not as stylish in the public clinic either, but they seemed much more in tune with their patients. Doctors' offices were computerized but still had some twenty-year-old furniture. The polyclinic in my old neighborhood in Vilnius, where I was a patient for eight years, looked better than it had on my last visit in 2001. The walls were painted in lighter colors and the building had new windows, though the same uncomfortable waiting-room chairs and old restrooms remained. It was, perhaps, less crowded than I remembered it.

On our way to the cafeteria at the university hospital, Lina, a cardiologist, shared her memories with me. "In the early nineties it was really tough here. We lacked everything—sheets, syringes, heating, medications. We asked patients to bring their own, so we could operate, keep working. Then things improved, but never to a satisfactory level. And now, with this crisis, again there are cuts, and we ask those who can afford it to pay for some supplies." The cardiology unit where Lina worked was completely updated with state-of-the-art technologies and laboratories. Lina commented that she felt more connected to the world of medicine now than she did years ago.

By contrast, the emergency room at the same hospital looked as if I had returned to Soviet times: the smell of the restroom, lack of toilet paper, and dark green walls all revived and sharpened my memories. Initially I had the thought that I would be scared to enter this emergency room as a patient. But after watching the staff work, I changed my mind. Lines moved smoothly. Although patients complained about wait times, most were seen in less than two hours. The head of the unit, a young, energetic, and enthusiastic woman in her thirties, took me outside and showed me an unfinished building. "We are waiting for this brand new and updated ER unit to finally be done." According to her, the 2008 crisis, which hit Lithuania particularly hard, had delayed the construction of the new building.

The state, both Lithuania and the EU, are the main drivers of health-care development. The Lithuanian Ministry of Health controls three university hospitals. Regional hospitals are controlled by local administrations. When Lithuania became a member of the EU in 2004, the state used the funding available through EU integration projects to update the health-care infrastructure, including technological upgrades. This influx of money coincided with the second stage of restructuring the health-care system.[22] Reform advocates no longer argued that private health care offered technological advantages. Their rhetoric shifted to expanding patients' choice of providers, disease prevention, and patient responsibility for health. The stated goal was to have 60 percent of primary health care in private hands by 2008. The National Health Insurance Fund was instructed to contract with private institutions (mostly primary care providers) to provide more choices for patients.[23]

By 2007, private practice accounted for only approximately 10 percent of health care, and none of the attempts to establish private hospitals as an alternative to public hospitals had been successful. In 2014, private hospitals still offered fewer than 1 percent of the hospital beds in Lithuania.[24] According to the doctors and nurses I spoke to, every news story that got traction in the national media was about long lines and informal payments. The suggested solutions were to privatize, freeze state funding, and improve managerial practices. The medical staff understood this pattern as a part of an organized effort to destroy (sužlugdyti) hospitals and polyclinics and then privatize them cheaply.

One of their concerns was that health care would meet the same fate as other privatized public goods, such as heating and electricity. In the late 1990s and early 2000s, municipalities signed long-term contracts that put public utilities into private hands. Instead of leading to greater efficiency and lower costs for consumers as promised, the change increased costs for the majority of the population. Folk-type conspiracy theories about the privatization of major hospitals animated the conversations and comments over coffee breaks about the state of health reform.

The Medical Gift Law

During the first stage of health-care reform there was an attempt to legalize informal payments through the Medical Gift Law. It decreed that doctors and health-care services administrators were not allowed to receive gifts, except symbolic ones (valued at no more than 1 minimal life index [*minimalaus gyvenimo lygio indeksas*], which at the time was 125 litai).[25] The law was abandoned in 2006 after debates in the parliament and criticism from nongovernmental organizations such as TIL. The doctors' union and the Ministry of Health had both supported the bill; the latter provided data showing that 95 percent of patients wanted to pay or give (*atiskaityti*) directly to doctors.[26] Opponents argued that the law legalized bribes and was undignified for both the patients and doctors because it effectively made payments or gifts mandatory. More important, opponents argued, the law did not increase transparency in the doctor-patient relationship. The debates reached their high point in 2004, when Lithuania became a member of the EU, filled with the zeal of Europeanization. According to some, the law was non-European because no similar law existed in any Western European country. Once the gift law was removed from the Civil Code, a new round of debates started about ways to refashion and codify informal payments and nontransparent income into formal, legal copayments.

The Medical Gift Law had the effect of transforming the little white envelopes from bribes into gifts. Its repeal effected another discursive shift, from the language and legal regime of gifts to the logic of transparency and copayments. This shift, in some ways, resembles controversies and changes in the market for human eggs analyzed by Catherine Waldby and Melinda Cooper. Previously, eggs were provided by volunteer donors through national donor registries and made available to women trying to conceive. Over time, however, these systems were superseded by a global market for human eggs, operating according to legalistic medical regimes. Supporters of the changes argued that the market system would increase the supply of eggs in response to demand. Contrary to predictions, the shift to a market did not improve the circumstances of the donors; rather, it led to exploitation and coercive labor relations. Waldby and Cooper (2008, 61) argue that recipients and donors are best protected by gifting systems when supply and demand for eggs are balanced. Their work shows the switching from the language of donations to the language of the market, as in the case of egg donors in IVF clinics shifts the larger discourse. I see the parallels in the discursive shift in the case of the Medical Gift law when the language of the market and payment prevailed over the language of donations.

In Lithuania, the cancellation of the gift law and orientation toward copayments marks a discursive shift from the system of donation to the logic of the market. This neoliberal opposition between informal/formal, nontransparent/transparent breaks down the particularity of doctor-patient relationship and connects it to privatized health care and formalized doctor-consumer relations. Meanwhile, the introduction of the logic of the market in health care opens up new possibilities for the expansion of health-care markets, with consequences (affordability, overtesting and overtreatment, medical debt) that may not necessarily dignify existing doctor-patient dynamics and medical encounters.

Economies of Care

By 2010 the number of private clinics had grown; roughly 25 percent of patients signed up for private primary-care clinics, which mostly offered family medicine, pediatrics, consultations with specialized doctors, diagnostic procedures, and outpatient surgeries. These institutions complained that the system of bribes and the culture of envelopes disrupted their business and precluded their growth. The managers of private clinics I interviewed voiced their disappointment that even though they paid taxes, they could not compete with the public hospitals for doctors and patients who were still enmeshed in the system of envelopes.

"It is absurd! To put bribes into doctors' pockets, in the twenty-first century! And the state does nothing. Even worse, they wanted to frame it as gifts," complained Andrius, the frustrated director of the private Neries Klinika in Vilnius. He ridiculed the enveloped practice: "How do I know how to give? How much to give? Is that too little or too much? It all causes anxiety. If you go through your networks, then you have to think how to thank them and not be in debt to your acquaintances." Meanwhile, in the private clinic, "it is very clear how much you have to pay. In fact, you can call in advance and ask, come, pay, and leave." Indeed, patients, caregivers, and medical personnel all reference the anxiety involved with enveloped practices, yet they continue to engage in them.

Andrius contrasted envelopes and payments as different sets of practices: envelopes were convoluted, requiring patients and caregivers to navigate complex, unwritten rules and social relationships, whereas payments were simple, equitable, rational, and clear-cut, involving no lingering debts or obligations. "You come, pay, and leave." Payments represent the world of autonomous subjects and a rationalized market for health care. This view obscures the complexities of how prices are set, what drives them, how the payment is produced, and what the patient has to do in order to make a copayment.

Most of the medical staff at the clinics worked under part-time contracts. Neries Klinika had contracts with eighty doctors; only eight of them were permanent, full-time employees. Andrius told me that it was hard for the clinic to meet doctors' full-time salary demands. Top doctors demanded 20,000–30,000 litai per month, claiming that this was the amount needed to match their current income from working at the public hospital, consulting at a private clinic, and from envelopes. The clinics could not offer such salaries because there were not enough patients using their services.

Neither Andrius nor the politicians and anticorruption officials accused the doctors of taking bribes; rather, they described doctors as hostages and victims of the system and its tradition of envelopes. The only way to expand private health care, they asserted, was by introducing official copayments and private insurance. Private clinic managers recommended that the state contract with them and divert part of the health-care budget to enable privately owned institutions to deliver some health-care services, and thus offer greater choice to the patients. Without such measures, they said, there was little hope of change: private clinics would depend on medical tourism and Lithuanians living abroad who returned to undergo medical procedures in their home country.

Despite the negative outlook of the clinic managers, private health care gained some ground. The clinics commissioned articles and advertised their services in magazines and newspapers. People from regional towns and the countryside often used consultations with specialists at private clinics as a way of gaining faster admission to university (public) hospitals. Many patients also appreciated the sleekness and faster service of private clinics. Young and middle-class patients often chose private clinics to avoid long lines when they did not have serious medical conditions.

Other patients at the private clinics felt ripped off and returned to public polyclinics and hospitals. Aida, a thirty-seven-year-old accountant from Vilnius, initially went to Neries Klinika to avoid long lines at the polyclinic. Aida spent close to a couple of thousand litai at the private clinic for tests and follow-up appointments. The tests were never ending, as she put it. When Aida was told her condition was precancerous, she realized that it would make more sense for her to switch to the local polyclinic, since she would become a chronic patient with gastroesophageal reflux disease and could not afford visits to the private clinic. She returned to the public clinic to see a gastroenterologist, taking an envelope containing 50 litai. At first, she recalled, she was not sure whether she would give the envelope to the doctor. "I was thinking, if I liked the doctor and would consider coming back, I'd give her that little envelope. The gastroenterologist was friendly, seemed competent, and explained everything better than the doctor at the private clinic, so I gave her the envelope when I was leaving. I know I will come back."

Some doctors shared these patients' views. I met family doctors who, after working for a while at private clinics, switched back to the public ones to avoid the pressure to sell tests. Loreta did so, she told me, because she wanted to be a doctor, not a salesperson. Other doctors at the public hospital thought private clinics were trying to attract patients who had money and then rip them off with unnecessary tests. In these cases, the doctors argued that the well-off patients would eventually come back to the public hospitals and change their perceptions about private institutions being better than public ones.

The private system, with its seemingly rational payment structure, and the public system, with its practices of informal payments embedded in social relations, mutual expectations, and responsibilities, represent two different economies. The envelopes are part of what anthropologists define as a human economy, in which money acts as a social currency to create, maintain, or sever relations between people rather than to purchase things (Graeber 2012, 158). It is an economy made and remade by people in their everyday lives (Hart, Laville, and Cattani 2010, 4). There is no definitive or stable way of calculating the value of exchanges or setting the amounts of money transmitted in envelopes, boxes of chocolates, or bags containing food or drink. This fluidity reflects the uniqueness of the individuals involved in the transactions and the diversity of the exchanges in which they engage. Aida's example shows how patients ground their decisions based on affective (bio)metrics, which is rooted in personal experience rather than on institutional status or assumed transparency of payments.

Andrius, the director of the private clinic, pointed to the anxieties the envelopes created: uncertainty about how much to give and the sense of obligation or debt that informal payments raise. However, as Jacques Godbout and Alain Caille point out, "The state of indebtedness is not intrinsically one of neurosis, and the goal is not to break free from it but to learn how to give in return, to play the game within this system without being taken advantage of" (1998, 40). Thus, while decisions about how much to give and how to offer it in a dignified way do cause anxiety, they also bring pleasure and gratitude. In the following chapters, I describe how patients spoke about being grateful to doctors and wanted their envelopes, gift boxes, and food items to be accepted. Doctors, too, worried about striking the right balance between being thanked and being bought, but they also described being moved by their patients' gratitude and the thoughtfulness of some of their gifts. Everybody played a game that was implicit and multilayered. Patients and caregivers entered and learned about the world of envelopes through stories, as well as through observing and participating in the actions of their grandparents, parents, relatives, and friends. These complexities and nuances signal a different economy of relations, driven by the will to care for oneself and the loved ones. This way of caring connects family members, friends, neighbors (including doctors) into caring collectives that work within the reality of envelopes blurring the boundaries of formal/informal spheres of life.

The Ambivalent State

Since 1990 every minister of health in Lithuania has walked a tightrope when discussing the issue of informal payments. Even if they define the transaction between the patient and the doctor as a bribe, they immediately qualify this definition by conceding that not all such transactions are bribes. On the one hand, officials acknowledge that Lithuanians want to thank their doctors, and this wish should be respected. On the other hand, the ministers condemn the extortion of money. State officials realize that the line between a gift and a bribe is a shifting one, drawn by the dynamics of each individual encounter. Universal rules or administrative measures are hard to apply. For instance, Minister of Health Algis Čaplikas, who was often praised by free-market advocates for his willingness to introduce copayments, stated in 2008: "The ideal scenario would be if we could replace unofficial payments with official copayments . . . though it's not clear yet how we will come to an agreement with doctors and society. A system that has existed for fifty years can't change in a day, we have to change ourselves."[27] The minister underlined that the practice is almost impossible to uproot without the collective agreement of all Lithuanians, not only doctors or state officials.

Managers of private health-care institutions and other experts have criticized public officials for sustaining the situation that makes envelopes neither legal nor illegal. Although informal payments are officially illegal, the state's responses are ambiguous. In 1998, when the practice of envelopes triggered police interest, a scandal erupted in Panevėžys and Vilnius. The weekly magazine *Veidas* reported on it in an article that began: "Every Lithuanian knows that it is appropriate to thank doctors by giving them money, flowers, and sweets." The article described the case of a woman from Vaivadų village, Jadvyga A., who complained to the police that at the municipal hospital in Panevėžys, four heads of the wards and one family doctor were taking bribes. The police started a sting operation. Marked money was found in doctors' pockets and wallets. The doctors' union reacted immediately by accusing the police of provocation and Stalinist techniques. The next day the attorney general dismissed the case.[28]

This case was unusual, but what is revealing about it is that it was the actions of the police that were defined as scandalous. It also speaks to the difficulty of dealing with the practices of informal payments through administrative measures.

Almost every month there is news in Lithuania about corrupt public officials being arrested. When I asked about legal proceedings against doctors, an official at the corruption prevention unit told me that it would be impossible to act because then every doctor should be arrested. In that case, he asked, "Who will treat us?" An administrator at a public hospital added: "Now we have to fight corruption. To me, it seems like the same as witch hunts in the Middle Ages or campaigns against enemies of the people in Soviet times. Nowadays, corruption is that enemy."

The state's ambivalence toward informal payments in health care is also useful in a way because it has allowed the state to keep the health-care system and its infrastructure functioning through years of transformation, while filling in the gaps of state apparatuses and institutional care. By accepting implicit norms and avoiding show trials, the state effectively acknowledges (like Lenin and Stalin in earlier times) that health care is local and operates based on logics that cannot be reduced to that of the market.

Health Care Cannot Be Free

The future of medicine in Lithuania must be market based, say various experts and private health-care managers, some politicians, and the media—all in unison. For instance, in 2010, the president of the Free Market Institute, Rūta Vainienė, who is also a member of the Bureau of Health-Care Reform (Sveikatos Reformos Biuras) and a leading expert on the issue, stated: "The Ministry of Health is treating medicine not as a business and a service to the client, but as a social function of the state. That is a deficient practice, and it shouldn't be this way. Because where there is money, the rules of the market and free competition should work." According to this health-care expert, current policies discriminate against private clinics, and legal copayments are necessary to eliminate the "deeply rooted tradition of envelopes."[29]

Since 2000, the notion of transparency emerged as a regulatory practice and a way of governing. One measure intended to increase support for a market-based health-care system was to make the current costs more obvious to citizens. Under the health-care law, the health-care tax was broken out as a separate item on payroll tax statements. In 2009, a separate health-care tax was levied, requiring both wage earners and the self-employed to contribute 72 litai per month (with the state making contributions to cover the unemployed, students, children, refugees, disabled people, and pensioners).

Additional mechanisms to increase transparency (including auditing and accounting measures, performance indicators, and quality standards) are seen as tools to increase the openness of health-care systems. Elsewhere in the EU, where prepaid universal health care is dominant, private companies and associations have been among the most active groups in the drive for transparency. In this sense, transparency is a coordination mechanism in markets under construction (like, for instance, health care) and a way to establish the rules of the game (Blomgren and Sunden, 2008: 1513).

The 2008–18 health-care reform projects focused on optimizing the hospital networks by merging smaller hospitals and strengthening regional and university hospitals. It also aimed to fundamentally change the way health care is funded by transforming informal payments for medical treatment into official copayments and introducing additional (voluntary) health-care insurance. The state will no longer invest directly in the health-care sector; care will instead be funded only by the health-care tax and private insurance. This shift in health-care funding is seen as "a tool to eliminate informal payments" and increase patients' responsibility for their health, thus reshaping patienthood in Lithuania. Therefore, the final stage of the health-care reform seeks to transfigure informal payments into copayments through the mechanism of transparency and by calculating the real costs of health care. The reforms had set a deadline of 2012 for the state to set prices for basic treatments (including a base price for the treatment, a facility's operating costs, financial costs, and so on) and make clear to the public the amount the state would contribute and the amount of the official copayments to be paid out of pocket or by private health insurance.

This final step has been stalled since 2009, although it has never been formally abandoned or reformulated. When the global financial crisis hit Lithuania in 2008, no political party dared to introduce copayments. Opinion polls showed that the majority of Lithuanians were against the plan.[30] Studies done by TIL revealed citizens' acquiescence with the system of informal payments, even when media stories reported that patients were paying more than 100 million litai out of pocket for medications, payments to private clinics, and fees for elective procedures at public health-care institutions.[31]

Supporters of reform often have stated in the media that patients do not understand that health care is not and cannot be free. Patients have been accused of false consciousness and irrationality for failing to recognize that envelopes are effectively the same as payments. They have also been accused of failing to take responsibility for their own health. One of the reasons for this attitude, it was argued, was free health care itself. This position is negated by the argument in favor of copayments, which holds that because people are already paying doctors, the payments simply need to become formal and transparent. Privatization advocates thus tacitly acknowledge that envelopes demonstrate patients' willingness to shoulder the cost of care, but not exactly in a neoliberal sense.

The discourse of responsibility, prominent in what is described as neoliberal governance, is not new to the former Soviet bloc nations (Collier 2012; Yurchak 2003; Zigon 2011). Responsibility is a value common to both neoliberalism and Soviet modernity. Stephen Collier argues that the values of socialist society continue to be reinscribed after the collapse of the socialist regime. Responsibility is an evident example of this reinscription. The case of enveloped practices illustrates the tensions around responsibility, as it attempts to redefine the very notion of it. The neoliberal responsibility related to the introduction of official copayments in health care comes up against the already-existing responsibility enacted by enveloped practices. Envelopes are an expression of the will to care that represent efforts by self-aware individuals to provide for their own well-being and that of their family members, relatives, and medical practitioners.

According to Jared Zigon (2011, 155), the cultivation of individual responsibility in Soviet modernity is tied to the ambiguity between the primacy of the collective and that of the individual. Precisely, this ambiguity might help strengthen individual responsibility. Similarly, Alexei Yurchak points out that during late socialism, meaningful individual responsibility was cultivated within one's intimate social network (Yurchak 2006, 109). However, this form of responsibility emerged much earlier; in fact, these preexisting practices only became visibly aberrant under socialism. The existence of enveloped practices of health care and their loose self-organization reveal gaps in the totality of state biopolitics. The discourse of neoliberal responsibility, expressed in the arguments for copayments, still struggles to reshape prevailing notions of responsibility related to health. It even intensifies personal responsibilities, adding layers to the practices and conduct of health and care rather than replacing existing perceptions.

Health-care experts advance arguments in support of transparency, the market, and the economy rather than care, rights, morality, or equality. In a way, enveloped practices have refused to be appropriated by the capitalist market. The repeated efforts by the media and state institutions, nongovernmental organizations, and international agencies to force enveloped practices to conform to the logic of the state and the market overlook the complexity of these practices, which sustain the existing model of public health care—a mixture of state funding and control coexisting with historically constituted social norms.

Money: The Same but Different

Health-care reform projects and policy studies define these enveloped practices uniformly as out-of-pocket spending that needs to be transparent and rational. Out-of-pocket expenses include the money spent on medications, herbal supplements, additional fees for elective tests, procedures at private clinics, and informal payments. It assumes that all moneys are equal. Following this logic, if the money is taken out of the envelope, paid through the cashier's office or bank, in an amount set by the market, the envelope becomes a payment, a dignified encounter.

From one perspective, envelopes and copayments might look like the same thing. Both involve transfers of money intended to improve well-being. Both are embedded in power relationships; they are neither fully transparent nor inherently moral. Yet they are not the same. To focus only on the money that passes hands, and to construct these two types of transactions as equivalent and interchangeable, is to miss the point. Anthropologists show how money is embedded in and constitutive of social relations, carrying different practical and moral forces as it moves through society (see Appadurai 1986; Guyer 1995; Lemon 1998; Martin 2015; Maurer 2006; Parry and Bloch 1989; Peebles 2013; Zelizer 1994). As Bill Maurer suggests, "Money may render everything calculable, but the systems of calculation and quantification on which it depends are not always as straightforwardly algebraic as one might imagine" (2006, 23). Money is relational (Zelizer 1997) and constituted ecologically (D'Avella 2014); different views of money are tightly linked to the ways in which we manage our ties with others (Dodd 2014, 291).

Copayments work within the logic of the market, modified to some degree by the state, the bureaucratic apparatus of a particular hospital, and the interventions of insurance companies. A payment is based on equivalences, whereby for a specific price one gets a specific service (Godbout 1998). For instance, surgery to remove a gallbladder or a malignant mole is assigned a value that emerges from obscure but supposedly rational calculations of costs (equipment, supplies, and medical and administrative labor, whose costs are, in turn, determined by the market). Payment is related to a particular medical procedure, and the personality/particularity of a doctor or a patient is not of primary importance in this formal payment relationship. The sum is visible, legal, and taxable. Hence, the payment is transparent in the sense that it is explicit.

The market principle in which copayments are grounded, however, is not necessarily produced by the social system (Laville 2010, 231). Neither is it simple, clear, or transparent. The Lithuanian patients I talked to were resistant to copayments partly because it was not clear to them how copayments would be calculated and whom they would benefit. Patients like Lucija suspected that hospital administrators and bureaucrats would benefit the most, not doctors or nurses. The system of payments seemed abstract and obscure.

The amounts that people place in envelopes are the result of complex negotiations, as this book will go on to detail, and each transaction is unique. The diversity and range of offerings for the same medical procedure differentiate them markedly from fixed copayments. Sometimes patients were not even certain they would give the doctor an envelope that was already sitting in their pocket. Envelopes are rooted in mutual expectations and obligations between patients and caregivers, on the one hand, and doctors and nurses, on the other. Patients and caregivers have expectations about their doctors and medical encounters. Their decisions about giving envelopes are based on whether these expectations are met.

Envelopes do not bring parity and equality between the patients and the doctors. Uncertainty, the absence of clear equivalences (how big of a smile one can get for an envelope), and the existing range of envelopes for the same procedures put the possibility of precise equivalences into question. In that sense, the envelope transcends the logic of the payment. Even if it might look like a payment, there are no clear equivalences, and it does not follow regulations or bureaucratic protocols. Envelopes bring personalities into professional relationships. They also generate ongoing feelings of entitlement and obligation. As the next chapter illustrates, many patients and their relatives told me that giving an envelope to a doctor made them feel free to come back and ask questions, make appointments, and arrange surgeries for their family members and friends. Doctors sometimes noted that their patients felt entitled to knock on their office doors to ask for help even though neither doctors nor patients considered each other to be friends. Thus, envelopes create a delicate web of obligations that is rewoven and renewed through a multitude of complex calculations based on experiences, anxieties, and diagnoses.

Enveloped practices invite a reconsideration of the idea of public health and the way good doctors should be rewarded, one that avoids a preoccupation with the logic of the gift or bribe. One way to think about this would be to adopt David Graeber's notion of "everyday communism," based on permanent mutual indebtedness: "a type of egalitarian society which is based neither in exchange nor in reciprocity—except . . . it does involve mutual expectations and responsibilities" (2012, 102, 121). Envelopes, too, could be defined as neither exchange nor reciprocity (or incomplete forms of exchange and reciprocity, in which everyone is aware of debt relations even if nobody is keeping ledgers).

The envelope system is pervasive in Lithuania, part of the fabric of society. Envelopes and the economy of relationships in which they are embedded resemble what Pierre Clastres (1989, 192, 199) defines as a subsistence economy: a market without surplus that sustains the society and not the state. A transformation from this relational logic to a market of regulated and codified copayments and of private capital investment and profits would upend Lithuanian health care. It is questionable whether such a regulated and transparent system would be more caring, egalitarian, or just, which, as we will see, is what everyone seems to want. In the meantime, the envelope system persists. To better understand the logic of enveloped care and how these practices have continued through major political, ideological, and economic shifts in Lithuania, we have to unravel how these implicit norms are shaped. In the chapters that follow, I explore how patients, caregivers, and medical practitioners encounter and participate in the enveloped economy of care.

Interlude II
THE SURPRISE

A man goes to a grocery store in Antakalanis, a neighborhood in Vilnius, where a large university clinic is located. He buys a box of chocolates and a bottle of sparkling wine. That night he goes to see his girlfriend and brings the bottle and the box to her place. They open the box of chocolates and find an envelope with 50 litai inside. . . . A friend of mine told me this story, which happened to his friend. The doctors at this clinic are swamped with boxes and bottles; one doctor had connections at the store, so he was able to take them there and exchange them for money. . . . That's why I always give envelopes.

This tale, recounted to me by Rūta, a forty-six-year-old secretary, is less common than the story of the traveling box, but it still circulates widely. The storyteller always explained to me that the doctor had connections in the store and returned the box for resale. The moral of the story is usually that what doctors really need is money, not chocolates—and that it pays to check the box carefully.

This second canonical tale about the box of chocolates introduces new elements: an opened box, a monetary gift, reselling, stores, and a person outside the doctor-patient relationship (the cooperative store clerk). The box no longer has a distinguishing mark; it is a commodity that can be resold. The box is opened and the money discovered not by the original giver but by a stranger.

Variations on this tale include the neighborhood and city where it happens and the gender of the protagonist. In addition, by specifying the amount and currency of the money (rubles, litai, or occasionally US dollars), the storyteller places the story in either the socialist or the postsocialist period.

Nothing else changes. It is always a young person who benefits from buying a box of chocolates. The recipient always knows immediately that the box

originally came from a doctor who failed to open it and find the gift. This knowledge connecting the doctor and the box is implicit. The recipient always keeps the
money and never considers returning to the store to report the find. The tale is
always set in Vilnius or Kaunas, the cities where large clinics and medical schools
are located. The box always bypasses its intended recipient. The doctor's personal
connection with the store owner or employee who accepts the box for resale is a
crucial element of the tale because the practice of returning products to a store
for a refund is not common in Lithuania.

Unlike the story of the circulating box, this tale does not posit a closed social
circle; on the contrary, it describes a network of exchange that extends to random
people. Moreover, it is a tale of consumption rather than of saving or recirculat-
ing goods. When I heard this story, other listeners usually debated the value of
the gift. They also discussed what the doctors do with the excess of chocolates,
alcohol, and sweets they receive. Do they need them? Would not it be better just
to slip an envelope into the doctor's pocket?

The doctor's failure to open the box or to realize that the box might contain
more than candy can be interpreted as evidence that the doctor does not expect
to receive envelopes. And a doctor who decides to resell a box of chocolates is
probably short on money. Thus, the tale and the listeners' comments tend to
encourage people to feel compassion toward doctors who lack money and to
offer envelopes instead of chocolates. This is also illustrated by another canonical
tale about a box of chocolates that is filled with money instead.

> Dr. Petras was an excellent doctor, loved by his patients and colleagues.
> One day he got a small box of chocolates from a patient for helping him
> fill out disability forms. The patient's short-term disability allowance
> was confirmed by the city medical committee. The patient came back to
> the doctor to thank him and gave him this box of chocolates.
>
> Dr. Petras put the box on the shelf and forgot about it. The following
> week the doctor was invited out to dinner. It was late in the evening and
> the stores had closed when Petras remembered the dinner and realized
> he didn't have anything to bring the hostess. Then he noticed the box of
> chocolates on the shelf. The doctor went to the dinner party and gave
> the chocolates to the hostess. When it was time for the dessert, the host-
> ess set the box of chocolates on the table and opened it, revealing a box
> full of money instead. Everybody at the table laughed. The next day the
> doctor told the story to his colleagues at the hospital.

I heard this tale from a doctor and a nurse. The doctor in the story was represented as someone who was no longer working or who had passed away. The
doctor-protagonist is represented as the original storyteller. As in the previous

two canonical tales, the doctor does not open the box himself. The new element in this version is the party guests who witness the hostess opening the box and thus seem to corroborate the truth of the narrative. The patient is absent from the scene. The box is always full of money.

I heard this story in 2009–10, though it most likely dates to the turbulent transition in the early 1990s. In the first years of Lithuania's independence from the Soviet Union, inflation had reached almost 1,000 percent per year. So, even a big chocolate box full of money did not necessarily represent a large amount.

These stories emphasize that the doctor really does not care about the contents of the box; he helps the patient without thinking about it. Either the doctors do not recognize that chocolate boxes might contain something else, or they are indifferent to both chocolates and money. However, these tales can also be read as illustrating the potential for miscommunication between doctors and patients. The fact that the doctors take the box at its face value means that they have failed to understand a subtle message from the patient and are indirectly punished for this lack of perception by forfeiting the hidden envelope with money. Doctors do not necessarily recognize patients' efforts to communicate things, so this also teaches patients not to assume that their efforts and signs of attention are received and understood. Finally, these stories question the rationale of giving and the effects of giving and receiving. Do the doctors care about their patients? Do they care what they receive from patients? These are fundamental questions in Lithuanian health care.

BEING CAUGHT
Envelopes and Illness

"I don't know where this knowledge comes from. It is somehow self-evident. It is like a norm—not mandatory, but it will be better for you. Probably better. Perhaps," said Rasa, a caretaker. Rasa's description of enveloped health-care practices reflects the views of many other patients and caretakers. The practice evolved many years ago, they concurred, yet no one could trace exactly when it started. It both is and is not mandatory; the delicate questions and dilemmas about whether to give an envelope, and when and how much to give, affect the lives of people who encounter illness in both abstract and practical ways. The envelope holds the potential to obtain better care and gives patients leverage over doctors, but it also causes anxiety and disappointment for patients and caregivers.

In interviews, patients and doctors often described giving envelopes as "something you can't escape," "a tradition," "a cult of giving," "a remnant of the Soviet past." In Lithuania, someone may be for or against the practice, but it is impossible to be unaware of the phenomenon. Their presence is signaled by the canonical tales about envelopes and circulating boxes of chocolates that people hear from coworkers, relatives, friends, and family members; by rumors; and by news outlets and social media. Once a family is touched by illness, they engage with enveloped practices more directly, deciding whether to give, or putting money in an envelope, perhaps with contributions from other family members or friends. Even preconceived notions about bribes and what counts as unacceptable behavior change when one is hit by a serious illness. The envelope becomes a force that, some believe, can transform doctors from rude, uncaring, and ill-tempered people into subservient subjects. It also exerts power over patients and relatives, who place their faith in its ability to bring about attentive care and healing. Thus, it symbolizes both good and bad care for the patients. However ambiguous, envelopes empower patients to face the uncertainty that comes with illness, and to not feel lost in the health-care system. They foster patients' and relatives' belief in successful surgeries and allow them to cope with complications as inevitable, rather than resulting from neglect by a medical practitioner. In this sense envelopes work as affective (bio)metrics based on a biographical understanding of life, where good care is measured by a singular experience of being cared for.

In this chapter I explore how practices of enveloped care are set in motion and how they order reality, beginning with health-care experiences during socialism that highlight the continuities with the informal economy of illness that prevails in the country. I present accounts I heard from informants about the practices of enveloped care, and I examine how patients and caretakers get acquainted with, perceive expectations around, and enact these practices. The informants' accounts of their relation to envelopes open up other relations. The stories I document here illustrate how complex these practices are. They expose anxieties about giving, illness, and caring. These accounts also reveal how enveloped practices relate to kin dynamics helping them to keep faith and accept fate. They also show how affective (bio)metrics work. By exploring the contradictory logic of giving and its limits, this chapter shows how an envelope becomes part of the healing process itself and a tool for coping with the limitations of biomedicine in Lithuania. The envelope has twofold efficacy: it helps people heal and ensures that Lithuania's particular health-care system and economy continue to function. In this way, everyone seems to be "caught" in the envelope, which can help us better understand how these practices endure despite deeply ambivalent feelings about them and repeated efforts to curtail them.

A Long Bus Ride and an Enduring Practice

In the mid-1970s, at the height of mature socialism when Soviet rule seemed interminable, Adomas was a teenager riding on a bus from the town of Balbieriškis to Vilnius with his mother. Three older men on the bus were loudly complaining that it was almost impossible to get good care without money, cursing greedy doctors. Adomas's mother—a teacher, activist, and communist believer—interrupted the older men: "What are you talking about? You yourselves are stuffing doctors with money and then complaining that they request money?" Her comment ignited a heated conversation throughout the whole bus, splitting the passengers into different camps: those for and against giving money, those who thought that doctors were to blame because they took the money, and those who thought it was the patients' fault for giving it.

Adomas, now in his early fifties, told me that it felt like a long bus ride. His mother explained to him later that these men had an outdated understanding of the system; they did not understand that health care was free in the Soviet Republic of Lithuania. She implied that giving envelopes to the doctors was a relic of prewar Lithuania. In other words, enveloped practices of care dated from the days when peasants and, later, farmers brought gifts and food to doctors instead of cash.

Medical care during the Soviet era reflected the regime's paternalistic approach to health and education. Both were structured as ways of disciplining and controlling the population (Verdery 1996). Despite limited treatment options, there was no shortage of doctors and no limit on hospital stays. With a diagnosis such as heart arrhythmia, a patient could stay in the hospital for two or three months. At the same time, the state retained strict control of medical knowledge and health care. Michelle Rivkin-Fish (2005, 26) points out that women patients constantly faced bureaucratic inconveniences and obstacles to obtaining care, which led them to describe health-care settings as factories. Health care in public hospitals became a deindividualizing "assembly line" (Taussig 1980). I heard several stories about health-care experiences during socialism: the difficulty of getting imported medications to treat serious illnesses; encounters with drunk doctors in hospitals and polyclinics; the rudeness of medical practitioners; and the "horse medicine" that was used to treat people.

Yet patients in Soviet Lithuania were autonomous in defining their medical problems. They could decide which specialist to see based on self-diagnosis. Moreover, because referrals from general practitioners were not required to see specialists, they could make their own decisions about which doctor to see though their choice was limited to the local polyclinics. If patients were not satisfied with local doctors and thought they lacked competence, they often used their social networks and envelopes to obtain better medical care. The function of the family doctor as the gatekeeper to specialized medicine was introduced only after the health-care reforms in the 1990s (Skultans 2006, 144).

As the previous chapter detailed, the debate over enveloped practices remains centered on the same questions that Adomas heard on the bus: some say that the doctors are provoking people into giving envelopes, while others argue that the patients are enslaved by outmoded, corrupt habits. The difference is that now, the prewar habits and practices of health care that Adomas's mother condemned as bourgeois have been redefined as Soviet. Informal knowledge, in the form of stories that circulate, provides a complex picture of health care. While it allows people to plot various scripts of medical encounters, it also pressures them to act.

Even if one regards informal payments as bribes, and doctors who accept them as corrupt, the emotional pressure to obtain the best care for one's self or loved ones might change or suspend these preconceived notions. That is how the will to care impels enveloped care.

Adomas's story not only provides a snapshot of experiences and perceptions of health care during socialism, but it also shows how notions of health care and actual practices of caring may be taken up and experienced differently when people confront the reality of serious illness. Adomas's mother had argued against envelopes, but when she needed care, her children and husband saw the envelope as a possible way to save her. In 1988, Adomas's mother, then sixty-two, developed a serious neurological illness, and it was then that he engaged with the debate on a personal level. His mother was losing her memory and cognitive abilities. (At that time, Alzheimer's disease was not a recognized diagnosis in Lithuania.) Doctors at the university clinic told the family there was not much hope. When Adomas, his father, brother, and sister-in-law gathered to discuss what to do, his sister-in-law said that they must give an envelope to the doctor. Maybe that would change something; perhaps there was some other treatment that they had not heard about. Nobody disagreed. During the discussion, Adomas got scared: "They were talking about the details, and I was thinking, oh God, will I have to do this? How will I do that? I began to run multiple scenarios in my mind." Luckily, his sister-in-law, who had been hospitalized multiple times and had also taken care of her parents, knew "how to deal with doctors" and volunteered to take care of the matter. When I talked to Adomas in 2009 and 2010, he laughed at how scared he had felt in 1988: "I was freaking out about becoming an adult." By the time we met, he had dealt with doctors and envelopes quite a few times, and he always faced the dilemma of whether to give and how much. With the help of his sister-in-law, he gradually became acquainted with the implicit norms and rituals of the practice.

Rasa: A Caring Daughter

"I am the one responsible for envelopes in the family," Rasa, a public employee, told me. I spoke with her when her mother was being discharged from the cardiology unit after a complicated heart-valve replacement operation. Rasa had been camping out at the hospital for the past three months; the heavy, dark circles under her eyes betrayed many sleepless nights. Before that, she had been taking care of her hospitalized father. Her aging parents had been in and out of the hospital for the previous ten years.

Rasa gathered information about doctors, hospitals, medications, diagnoses, and treatments. Her contribution to the family economy was to take care of her parents. She and her sister alternated the responsibilities of preparing food and spending nights at the hospital. Their brother was the major financial contributor. Rasa told me that she and her siblings always discussed how much money to give to the doctors, and her parents always asked whether the children had "settled accounts with the doctors."

"I thought I would go crazy when I had to do it for the first time, and my mother kept asking me whether I'd settled things with the doctors," Rasa remembered. "My mother walked by the doctor in the corridor of the unit where she was hospitalized, and the doctor didn't smile at her; she immediately called me to hurry up and bring gifts. My sister was skeptical. She thought that our mother was spoiled and was making things up." Nevertheless, the siblings agreed to give the doctor an envelope. Although Rasa had received advice from a coworker whose mother had been hospitalized for a similar condition in the same unit, she told me she felt anxious as she waited for the right moment. "See, you can't give too much or too little," she explained.

Since then, she has learned more about how to give. "The most important thing is to preserve your dignity and that of the doctor. I tell them that I understand how difficult their work is and what it means to work for a state institution because I work for one, too. Or I craft some kind of story, like, this is from my mother or my brother, and they would feel insulted if you don't take it. Or it's from a trip abroad. It depends. Sometimes I add a chocolate box or a bottle of wine. I think envelopes alone are too banal." All this happened, according to Rasa, in a "dignified way, saving face" (*išlaikant veidą*), "not buying" the doctor, and acting "as if nothing happened."

Rasa interprets the practice of enveloped care as a matter of dignity, saving face, and showing faith in the world of care. She expresses solidarity with the doctors, acknowledging their material needs and their hard work. Her empathy is not exceptional. Many patients and caregivers commented to me that the doctors were worthy of being rewarded for their care. Rasa described the doctors' responses: "Good doctors always say no, you have a lot of expenses . . . drugs are expensive." The worst thing, according to Rasa—and echoing Lucija—is when the envelope is refused; either there is no hope, or you gave it the wrong way.

At the same time, her envelope goes beyond pleasing doctors; it is interwoven with Rasa's parents' and their doctors' recognition of her as a caring person. Rasa started crying when she talked about the doctors who recognize that she "really cares" about her parents: "I will say that the good doctor acknowledges that I care for my parents . . . and only then takes an envelope." It is important for both her parents and their doctors that Rasa be a good daughter and caring person, which means expressing that care for her aging parents through material means. I asked whether her mother detected changes in the doctor's behavior after the envelope had been offered. "When she was discharged from the unit, the doctor hugged and kissed her. She was in heaven," Rasa told me with a big smile. Both Rasa and her mother want to be recognized as people, not only as patients or caregivers. The envelope has the power to make this happen.

Being Caught: The Force of Relations

While observing the interactions between patients and medical staff at the hospital, I often heard "talk to the doctor" (*pasikalbėti su gydytoju*) as a response to questions about future surgeries, medications, and treatment. For instance, if a nurse told a patient or a caretaker, "go and talk to the doctor" or "you need to talk to the doctor," it could mean "arranging an envelope." Some of the talks that I observed indeed meant talking and nothing else, while at other times, it perhaps meant the inclusion of an envelope. In my own history as a patient and a caretaker for my mother in the late 1990s and early 2000s, I remember being advised "to talk," but I interpreted it as referring to a verbal rather than a financial transaction, though perhaps I had misunderstood it at the time.

In this context of ambiguity and coded meanings, gestures, actions, and words were subject to multiple interpretations. A doctor's refusal to accept an envelope could be read as a sign that there was no hope for the patient, or simply that the offering was not necessary. The same interpretive methods were applied to the doctor's appearance, tone of voice, and facial expressions. If a doctor did not respond to a smiling patient, was she tired, focused on an important task, or simply indifferent to the patient's welfare? If the doctor wanted to talk to a patient on the eve of a surgical procedure, was he coming to discuss the procedure, or did he expect to receive an envelope?

The envelope became an explanatory framework for patients and caretakers. Surrounded by stories and rumors about envelopes that often contradict one's personal experiences, actors in medical encounters can see things that might otherwise be explained differently. If words and actions are subject to interpretation through the lens of the envelope, the reality of health care shifts. The envelope, and the language and actions associated with it, might be viewed as a form of a spell. In her ethnographical study on witchcraft in western France in the late 1960s, Jeanne Favret-Saada (1981) explores practices and beliefs among farmers. Viewing witchcraft as a symbolic system with social and psychological effects, she shows how farmers invoke it in their interpretations of misfortunes and social relationships, even though they might claim not to believe in the supernatural.

The language of the spell is employed to explain repeated misfortunes that occur without apparent reason as the work of a "force." Those who are caught in spells interpret language differently and speak differently (Favret-Saada 1981, 15, 17).

Lithuanian patients and caregivers are being caught in the field of the envelope after listening to stories of coworkers, parents, friends, and relatives. They are also inhabited by the language and practice of envelopes. When someone encounters an illness, questions like, "Should I give an envelope?" and "Am I being asked for an envelope?" cross their mind. By dealing with these dilemmas of giving or not giving, even if for just a split second, one is enveloped in the world of the envelope. Envelopes affect interpersonal relationships and events. Stories about envelopes are enacted in people's lives.

Being caught in the envelope also entails being caught in the network of relations centered on the envelope. Relations between family members, friends, other patients, as well as previous relations with doctors and nurses have their hold at the moment of illness and are present in medical encounters. This mindset leads people to see a chain of cause and effect that reinforces the power of the envelope. Being caught in the envelope allows one to see a series of provocations and repetitions that link the fate of treatment and protection against medical mistakes to the envelope. Here the envelope emerges as a play of forces, "a system of positions," as Favret-Saada (1981) calls it, which pressures an individual into a certain position. For instance, Rasa enacts her kin obligations by giving an envelope to the doctor for her ailing mother. Doctors are also forced into the position of implicitly or explicitly asking for envelopes, and patients into appearing eager to give. The envelope dictates the relationships and actions of all those who encounter it.

Begging White Pockets: Power and Provocation

Walking her dog after dinner on a Sunday night, Dalia, a forty-three-year-old secretary in a private company, felt an acute pain in her back. She took pain relievers, but the pain only got worse. After three hours, Dalia, who shares an apartment with her retired mother, could not bear the pain anymore and called an ambulance. An emergency nurse suspected a kidney stone or gallstone. Dalia gathered her passport, Social Security ID card, and wallet before she was taken to the emergency room of the university hospital.

Because Sunday nights are usually calm in the emergency room, Dalia was seen quickly. The doctor came in and ordered tests—blood, urine, and ultrasound—to confirm his diagnosis of a gallstone. She received intravenous painkillers and was transferred to the abdominal surgery unit. It was a sleepless night. The nurse on duty came by often to check on her and give her additional painkillers.

In the morning, the doctor who had admitted her to the hospital told her that she would need surgery once the inflammation had subsided within the month. "I didn't like his voice. He seemed rude, the way he told me about the surgery," Dalia told me the day after she got back from the hospital. She decided to choose a surgeon whom two other women in her hospital room had been talking favorably about and to offer an envelope. "But the nurse seemed nice, so I asked her what she thought about the other surgeon. The nurse told me, 'If I were you, I would stick with this one. Not all first impressions are right. He is a very good surgeon, a bit strange but good.'" Dalia decided to stay with the same doctor. I asked her whether she doubted him or whether she had been "provoked" on Sunday night at the ER. She looked surprised by my question and said: "I was in pain, I don't remember anything. It didn't matter then."

Patients who were caught by the envelope often talked about "provocation" and "being provoked." Examples of provocation included the doctor's tone of voice, a grim expression, paying too much attention to a patient's history, sitting too close, unfriendliness, and asking too few or too many questions. Some patients also referred to inanimate provocations, such as slow printers and computer connections, or the conspicuous pockets of the doctor's white coat, as signs that they should give envelopes. Describing the contact between the weak and the strong (bewitcher and bewitched), Favret-Saada observes that "whether it operates through speech, sight, or touch, [it] provokes a loss of force or of wealth" (1981, 112).[1] Similarly, a "strong" doctor may provoke a "weak" patient to give an envelope. Provocation, as experienced and reported by patients, describes a set of relations and obligations that come into existence upon contact with the doctor.

On the day of her discharge from hospital, Dalia recounted:

> He [the doctor] asked me to come to his office to talk, to get my sick-leave slip and prescriptions. My mother, who had visited me, told me that when I scheduled the surgery, I had to arrange things with him and give him an envelope. My mother always does that. I thought I would see how it went. I had the envelope with 100 litai in my pocket and went in. He told me to sit down. Then he pulled his chair closer to me. He talked slowly—asked whether I understood and agreed to have the gallbladder removal surgery. I said yes. "OK," he said slowly and took out the calendar. Very slowly. "Let's see," he said, "what we have got here . . . the earliest possible date is in three weeks. Is that OK?" he asked. What was this? I thought. I said OK . . . what else could you say? He gave me prescriptions, told me to see my family doctor, and gave me the list of tests that needed to be done before the day of the surgery. He wrote on a piece of paper what to do how many days before the surgery. "You also need the sick-leave slip, right?" he asked me again. Awkward—he

knew that I needed it. Then he slowly, again, put the paper in his printer and filled the form on his computer. The printer was incredibly slow. I think he was waiting for me to give money to him. The large pocket of his white coat was wide open before my eyes as if it was looking at me, begging me. Maybe, I think, he sat conveniently so that the pocket would face me. I don't know. Perhaps, Rima, you would have done differently, I don't know, but I put the envelope into that big pocket.

"What happened next?" I asked her. "The printer started working," Dalia smiled. "Maybe it was a coincidence or maybe not, but he hugged me, shook my hand, told me to take good care of myself, and that he would see me in three weeks. 'I bet you look forward to it, of course,' I thought, laughing to myself." She explained to me that giving him the envelope was like insurance. She hoped the surgeon would remember her when she returned for the surgery.

When do situations of provocation arise, and how are they recognized? Initially, Dalia was disinclined to offer the doctor an envelope. She felt provoked first by the suggestion "to talk," then from the apparently deliberate slowness of the doctor's movements and speech, and finally from the sight of his gaping pocket. All these phenomena have alternative explanations: perhaps the doctor was just tired or a naturally slow speaker. The delay in printing Dalia's sick leave slip could be readily explained by the limitations of the hospital's computer system, which is connected to the national social security database. Nevertheless, Dalia felt provoked. With her knowledge of the stories and rumors about envelopes and her mother's experiences, Dalia interpreted the encounter with the doctor before leaving the hospital through the lens of the envelope. This interpretation made her feel justified in giving him one, but she was not brimming with gratitude for the doctor, who struck her as good but also strange.

Symbolic objects and actions—the printers, pockets, envelopes, slowness, hallways, outcomes—appear to have interrelated effects. Patients seemed to test the boundaries of provocation as if it were a game in which the doctor and patient switch sides. As it did for Dalia, responding to a provocation can give a patient some sense of agency and control in facing an otherwise uncertain future. In this way, the envelope becomes a powerful force related to fate and faith in the future while also empowering the giver.

"I Gave the Envelope . . . You Will Recover"

Perhaps the envelope works like a placebo or the inverse of a placebo. Although the patient gives it to the doctor, it benefits the patient. Likewise, it does not offer an ethnomedical treatment, nor is it a substitution for a biomedical procedure

(Kleinman 1983; Moerman 2002). The envelope operates alongside biomedical notions of body and health. It strengthens the faith of relatives and patients in doctors and their treatment plans. The act of appeasing doctors fosters the patients' belief in a successful surgery and fast recovery. Therefore, the envelope, like a placebo, produces anticipated effects. Moreover, when complications such as pain and dizziness are explained in relation to the envelope, it becomes part of the healing process. Conversely, the belief that if you do not pay, you do not recover also circulated as rumors or horror stories.

The power of the envelope was often demonstrated with stories about anesthesiology. Unlike surgeons, anesthesiologists do not work in the units where patients are hospitalized, and so patients usually do not meet them until shortly before their surgeries. This makes arranging envelopes for anesthesiologists more complicated. An anesthesiologist's visit on the eve of surgery is often interpreted as an orchestrated means of collecting the envelope. According to many patients, however, the anesthesiologist's role is less critical than the surgeon's, so it is not life threatening if an envelope cannot be arranged.

The effects of anesthesia and recovery from it is the first thing that patients and caretakers experience or observe after surgery. Obviously, these depend on calculations of body mass and dosage; but the aftereffects, such as sickness and dizziness, were explained by the absence of an envelope, or the envelope's being too thin or too thick. In 2009, Adomas was taking care of his daughter, who had to undergo knee surgery. He gave an envelope to the surgeon, but he could not find the anesthesiologist and did not have the chance to give him anything. When Adomas's daughter felt sick after the surgery, he told me he thought it was because he had missed the anesthesiologist.

Another informant, Brigita, had thyroid surgery in 2005. At the time, she was living in a house with a leaking roof and a broken heating system, and her aunt arranged things for her. She asked her friends, relatives, and neighbors for information, went to see the doctor, chose the surgeon, and selected the date of the surgery. On the evening before the surgery, Brigita's aunt told her, "Don't worry, my dear, sleep well tonight, I gave the envelope, everything will be just fine. You will recover very fast." But Brigita felt sick after the surgery. "I vomited my guts out," she said, "I thought my aunt forgot to give the envelope to the anesthesiologist."

Five years after her first thyroid surgery, lumps in her thyroid were detected again, and in 2010 she returned for another surgery. This time, wanting to be sure things were done properly, Brigita decided to take care of everything herself. She gave an envelope containing 100 litai to the anesthesiologist. Her surgeon, the one who had operated on her five years earlier, refused to take money. Her aunt told me that "he was the honest doctor, he saw that she was poor." According to

Brigita, this time she recovered faster. "I felt sick, but not like the last time. No comparison, but I was vomiting. Yeah, maybe it was too much, the amount in the envelope, or maybe I can't stand these drugs." Like other patients, she had assumed that the money in the envelope would ensure successful healing, only to realize that the relationship between money and recovery is not straightforward. A thicker envelope does not guarantee freedom from side effects.

Rasa, the expert on the informal economy of illness, also interpreted her mother's slow recovery after her first surgery in relation to the envelope she gave the anesthesiologist. "I think I gave too much, so he was overgenerous with the anesthesia. She had hallucinations." A couple of years later, when Rasa's mother had to undergo complicated heart surgery, Rasa approached the anesthesiologist to give him an envelope. According to Rasa, the doctor told her: "I am superstitious. This surgery is very difficult; it might have complications. I can't accept this."

"I thought, that's it, my mother will die, and started crying," Rasa told me. Luckily, her mother recovered after a hospital stay of a few months. Rasa could not find the anesthesiologist. She saw him once and had the money, but she did not give it to him because she did not have an envelope to put it in. "I still feel the weight of it on my chest, that I didn't thank him. I am superstitious, too." But then she dismissed her belief: "I know it's nonsense." In the summer of 2010, however, her mother ended up in the ICU again. Rasa's superstitious fears were realized. "I was thinking, going through the past events . . . you know, getting crazy . . . and I thought that it was a series of misfortunes because I didn't thank the anesthesiologist or the doctor who found a defect in my mother's heart. Maybe it is just a coincidence."

Giving an envelope allows the giver to believe that everything will be OK. A caregiver may reassure a patient: "You can calm down; I gave the envelope. You will recover." Thus, the envelope functions as a mediator or a bewitcher, in Favret-Saada's words, producing the anticipated effects. If the outcome is bad, the envelope can be invoked to interpret medical mistakes and complications as unavoidable and bearable rather than malicious. In other words, the envelope has efficacy; it is a tool that patients use to relate to and collaborate with health practitioners, to have a hand in the complex clinical processes that are generally beyond a patients' expertise.

Other scholars have noted the effects of a belief in magic in other clinical settings. Writing about health care in modern China, Judith Farquhar and Lili Lai observe, "No matter how often we decry the 'dehumanizing' and 'objectifying' tendencies of contemporary biomedical clinics . . . amidst all the overlapping contingencies of illnesses and the inevitable ruptures between cause and effect, magical healing takes place" (Farquhar and Lai, 2015, 391). Decades earlier,

Marcel Mauss also observed that the medical profession has magical attributes: "Their skills go hand in hand with magic, and in any case their use of such complex techniques makes it inevitable that their profession should be considered marvelous and supernatural" ([1950] 2001, 36). Claude Lévi-Strauss observed that both shamanistic and psychoanalytic healing modalities depend on the power of the patient's belief in the efficacy of the practice (Lévi-Strauss 1963). He noted, "The therapeutic value of the cure depends on the actual character of remembered situations" (Lévi-Strauss 1963, 202). In part, the power of belief that the envelope will ensure a successful surgery and recovery in the biomedical context is similar to shamanistic and psychoanalytic sites.

A belief in the power of the envelope is not inherently at odds with a belief in medical knowledge. Belief is not lesser than knowledge; rather, it is a practice that produces reality. It represents a belief in both biomedicine and the power of good relationships to elicit the best medical practices. It is pragmatically located in social relationships and illness experiences (Good 1994, 23), where the symbolic and the scientific go hand in hand. Within this set of relationships, the envelopes act as enhancers of technology and surgical procedures and an expression of affective (bio)metrics marking best possible medical care as a subjective experience of being cared for.

The Power of Not Giving

"I always give, always pay," said Brigita, as we sat on a worn red couch in her living room on a cold Saturday in October. She had generously made time to talk to me between her daily chores of feeding pigs and milking cows. "Always?" I asked her. "Always. I mean, according to the situation," she answered. She did not seem to notice her contradiction. She described the provocations doctors employ: reviewing a patient's history for too long, asking too many questions, "wasting time and bullshitting and waiting to be bribed."

"Sometimes I think there is no need to give, but maybe not . . . maybe there is," Brigita slowly articulated her thoughts. She sounded uncertain. In the spring, Brigita had experienced sharp lower back pain and had an urgency to urinate. She suspected kidney stones. Brigita went to her family doctor, who ordered blood and urine tests and an ultrasound. She was sent for a consultation with a urologist at the same polyclinic. Before going into the doctor's office, she had prepared two envelopes. "I put 50 litai into one pocket and 100 litai into the other. I thought I would give depending on the results. It might be something serious," she explained. The doctor told her that she had a kidney inflammation and would have to take antibiotics and come back for a follow-up the next week.

Brigita reasoned, "It is only inflammation—you can't die from it. I could buy antibiotics for myself, so why give them envelopes if you don't have a serious illness? No reason, really. I left with both envelopes in my pockets. You don't give in such cases. No illness, no money. I will simply buy medication, and the inflammation will go away." She qualified her opinion: "Of course you ask around to find out what others are giving, but you act according to the situation: is it worth it, and can you afford it?"

Inflammation was a plausible diagnosis, and as long as Brigita felt she could take care of herself, she resisted paying the doctor. The diagnosis of an easily treated condition also implied that her interaction with the urologist might be limited to one or two appointments; hence there was no reason to nurture the relationship with the doctor. "What about your family doctor?" I asked. "Oh, the family doctor—sometimes I give her chocolates, and sometimes I add 20 litai to the chocolates. Not always, but she is the family doctor. It's different. Maybe she will prescribe me better medications."

Such decisions are not always arrived at so rationally. "Sometimes you lose your mind," Brigita confessed. When she was twenty-six years old, she recounted, she had a miscarriage. She was home alone. She called an ambulance, which took her to the hospital. The obstetrician was a nice old man. When she was on the operating table, she insisted on putting money into his pocket. "That was different. On the way to the hospital I lost my mind. I don't know why I got this idea. I was very scared. I was afraid that I would not be able to have kids. I thought, if I gave money to the doctor, I would be able to have kids in the future. I had this belief. I think he would have done everything all right anyway, honestly. . . . Thank God he took it. He didn't want to, but I insisted. I can't explain to you what got into me." Here, the situation and the envelope were linked to Brigita's future. What she defined as "losing her mind" was surrendering to the power of the envelope.

"If I hadn't had money, I would have told the doctor, I don't have anything to give you, do whatever you must do to me, cut me/kill me (*papjauti*)."

"Have you ever had to say this?" I asked her.

"No, but at the university hospital, in the same room with me, there was this woman who was from a village nearby; she had four kids and an alcoholic husband who had left her. She told the doctor, 'I don't have the money, I can't give you anything, do whatever you can (*kaip padarysit taip bus gerai*),' and guess what, they did a very neat surgery, and she got IVs, everything. I think they cared for her very well." With this story, Brigita seemed anxious to differentiate herself from the other patient, portraying herself as capable of giving and of taking care of herself. At the same, she seemed to be impressed by the treatment the other woman had received despite not giving anything.

Then Brigita told me another story she had heard about a different woman who, on explaining that she had no money, was told to borrow it. The woman had to leave the hospital and find another doctor. Being poor was no excuse for not giving anything. Having to borrow money or go into debt for treatment seemed terrifying to Brigita, as it did for most Lithuanians. I have heard other similar horror stories, but I could not find anyone who had personally been turned away from the public hospital and told to borrow money.

For Brigita, being unable to offer the doctor an envelope was an unfortunate situation that she felt fortunate to be able to avoid. Yet she had already envisioned herself being in this type of a situation. Her calculations about giving, contingent on multiple factors—the nature of the illness, her financial situation, the actions and situations of fellow patients, and the medical encounter itself—are shaped by the belief in the power of envelopes. She always gives, she says, yet she is reluctant to engage in the practice, except in a very emotional and stressful situation. The contradictions and inconsistencies in Brigita's attitude reveal enveloped care as something always in process and never predetermined. It shows how ambivalence is embodied in enveloped care.

Occasionally, enveloped practices reach their limits: patients and their caretakers refuse to give. To withstand provocations—grim faces, staring contests, brusque treatment, slow computers, or reminders of their previous encounters—they employ a range of techniques. Patients may go empty-handed to the first meeting with a doctor, inform doctors upfront that they do not have anything to give, raise their voices, create drama, or invoke their legal rights. In such exchanges, the envelope, although absent, remains a force.

Emilija, an opera singer, never gives envelopes. She has developed alternative strategies for obtaining satisfactory care. "I have never given a bribe or passed money in the envelope, and I have fifteen years of experience dealing with doctors. I took care of my mom, I buried my two brothers, and just recently my mother-in-law," she told me confidently and expressively as we sat in the backyard of her vacation home in a small town in the summer of 2010. "I belong to the category of people who can be angry. I demand things and raise my voice. I make fake phone calls. I create drama and stage a nervous breakdown. I try to speak their language," Emilija declared in a high-pitched voice, "usually, I get what I want."

The previous winter, Emilija had been a patient in the ear, nose, and throat surgery unit at the university hospital. She was placed in a room with three beds. In the beginning, Emilija and one other woman shared the room. On Sunday night, a third patient was admitted for a surgery scheduled for Monday morning. Emilija recounted, "She said hello, and her next sentence was a question: 'Who is your doctor? Do you know how much you have to give for the surgery?' I was shocked that people wanted to give money before the surgery. And everybody asks these questions!" Emilija continued in a dramatic voice:

> The women started to talk. This woman from this room gave this amount, and that one gave this amount. But I said there is no need to give. I asked this young woman, a basketball coach: "Why give? Is your surgery planned?" She answered, "Yes, it was scheduled a month ago." If the surgery is planned, you don't have to give anything. If you got here through your networks, they admitted you ahead of time; if the doctor is saving your life, then yes, you have to thank them. But if you waited for three months, then no way. None of us had any complications, and the doctor came to talk to us. I am telling you, people are spoiling our doctors.

She also told me that in the end, the coach did not give anything.

Emilija elaborated on her approach during medical encounters. "I never imply, show, or nod that I will be grateful. On the contrary. I show my knowledge and rights. I don't care about the grim faces. I can make grimmer ones. I don't think that the doctors will do something wrong to you purposely if you are following their instructions. I do imagine that some things would be faster if you gave." Emilija understood enveloped practices and was good at manipulating and subverting them. One time she took her mother to the emergency room because she suspected a heart attack. There she was told that her mother was experiencing an asthma attack. "It looked like asthma, but I knew it was the heart. I did not agree with them and demanded an EKG. They did it. I was right. They gave injections and medications. Then they told me there were no beds in the hospital, so I should take my mother home. I said that I would not take her home in such a condition and started making fake phone calls in this very dramatic tone. You know, I know how to act. After a while, when it was clear that we were not going to go anywhere, they found a bed—in another unit, but they did."

Emilija was not the only person I met who was skilled at creating drama. While observing patients and their relatives in the emergency room, I witnessed several dramatic scenes—caretakers refusing to take their relatives home, older patients demanding to be seen by older doctors rather than young residents, patients threatening to bring in journalists or boasting about relationships with powerful politicians, and sometimes patients insulting doctors openly. If someone, like Emilija's mother, was admitted to the hospital when there was a shortage of beds and others were being turned away, their relatives would tell me, "It's because of money; you have to write about this."

The medical staff I observed and spoke with hated the drama and tried to do everything according to medical protocols. Doctors and nurses tried to pacify angry relatives and patients because, according to them, anger was contagious. In some cases, the patients were transferred to other hospitals. Sometimes they calmed down or changed their minds after treatments took effect, or a bed was found for a dissatisfied patient in another unit. When the relatives or the patients threatened to complain to the director of the hospital or the minister of health, nurses or doctors would often bring them a form to fill out and say, "Please do."

Despite Emilija's personal opposition to giving envelopes, when her mother was in the hospital, Emilija's sister gave the doctor an envelope. "I couldn't convince her," Emilija told me. "Paying *before* is bad; I don't have an opinion about *after*." She paused, then said, "Maybe after a surgery or a treatment everyone could thank the doctor according to their financial abilities." Although Emilija eliminates actual envelopes from her medical encounters, she employs other affective tools to engage with the health-care system, such as her strong voice, acting abilities, and knowledge of medical language. She tries to rationalize the system by following the rules that she thinks are fair. Yet she, too, is caught in enveloped care: she cannot prevent her sister from giving an envelope on behalf of their mother, and she admits that she is not opposed to thanking doctors after surgeries or when they save patients' lives.

"I Would Have No Heart"

At the opposite end of the spectrum from Emilija was Justinas, who not only gave envelopes to his doctors but criticized patients who did not. "Tell me: how could I not thank the man who spent six hours on my heart? How? I would be heartless (*beširdis*)," he said, playing on the double meaning of the word. A retired ship mechanic in his late sixties, he was still working at a preschool as a handyman. Dressed in a dark blue working coat over a thick gray wool sweater and blue jeans, he sat in front of me in his small workshop in the basement of the preschool.

Justinas has been seeing his cardiologist regularly and has undergone two cardiac surgeries. In December 2009, Justinas had heart valve replacement surgery at the university hospital. On the eve of the surgery, the surgeon came to talk to him. "He sat on my bed, and we talked about life. He explained the surgery to me. He drew on a piece of paper how the mechanism would work. I told him frankly, 'Doctor, I want to thank you,' and was reaching for the envelope with 400 litai in it. He stopped me and said, 'If you want to thank me, you can do it after the surgery.' I said, OK. I understand, the surgery is difficult, anything could happen, I thought. I asked him: 'Doctor, what about an anesthesiologist, should I look for him before I go in?' He said, 'You know, it's not important, it's up to you.'" Justinas decided to thank the anesthesiologist after the surgery but could not find him later.

"I think that when I give after the surgery, it's a pure thank you," said Justinas, and told me about the patient with whom he had shared a room during his last surgery. "He was so stingy. We talked; he told me that he wouldn't give anything. When the staff suggested he buy extra medication instead of the basic ones, he always said that he could not afford it. He got everything. For free. He even dared to ask me what I received that he didn't. I think it's about honesty. You must have no heart if you don't thank the doctor who spent six hours on you, cleaning your clogged arteries and repairing your heart. It's not a car. Of course I will thank the doctor. He had my life in his hands. I must thank him. I am not a pig," Justinas said passionately. I asked him what if his roommate had indeed been poor. "No, he was also a mechanic. He lives in the neighborhood. They drive good cars. Just stingy. Stingy and heartless." The patients I interviewed usually talked about the honesty or dishonesty of doctors, but Justinas applied this criterion to patients, condemning those who gave nothing as dishonest. He was not alone. Quite often, patients felt pressured to give not by the medical practitioners but by other patients.

Justinas, like other patients who underwent complicated surgeries or long treatments, talked about his doctors favorably, emphasizing his own gratitude and intentions. Employing the language of reciprocity and the gift, they referred to the envelopes as a "sincere thank you" (*tikras atsidėkojimas*) and "payback." "I know when you don't have to give anything to the doctors," Justinas said with a playful smile.

"When?" I asked him.

"When you are healthy," he replied, laughing at his own joke.

Justinas told me that when he goes to meet a doctor for the first time, he goes empty-handed. "I don't have any bags with me. I don't want doctors to be distracted by what I might give to them. I want them to focus on me." But with a doctor he knows and defines as "almost a good acquaintance," Justinas behaves differently. He gives envelopes containing 50 litai to the family doctor and his cardiologist. "It's not a bribe. I know them. It is a thank you," he told me. Every Christmas and Easter, Justinas buys postcards and asks one of the teachers with good handwriting to write a card for his doctor. "I am bad with words," he explains. He adds 25 litai to the card for the nurse, too. "They tell me, 'Thank you! Thank you! But there is no need! Why are you doing this? You might need this to buy drugs, Justinas, you are not a banker.'" But he is firm: "I want to give them even more," he says proudly. He keeps giving the same amount every year because though he is not rich, he is not heartless, either. The envelopes are expressions of the will to care; Justinas cares about the doctors and himself.

Bribing God

When Aida, Adomas's daughter, started suffering from knee pain, he took her to a private clinic. "I didn't have time to schedule appointments or wait in line with her," he explained to me. Officially, Adomas paid 200 litai for the surgeon's consultation at the private clinic, where he told them Aida needed surgery. "He gave me his phone number at the public hospital, where he worked, so I could call him and arrange things." Adomas called the doctor, went to see him, and got a referral to the hospital. A few days later, his daughter went in for surgery. "Of course, I understood that I needed to give an envelope, even though the doctor didn't ask. But it was clear. At the private clinic I would have paid a minimum of 800 litai for the surgery alone, plus additional costs."

Adomas asked his sister-in-law and his girlfriend to help him to decide how much to put in the envelope. He also asked his colleagues whether they knew someone who had had similar surgery. He explained how he eventually decided on an amount between 300 and 400 litai. "I was getting numbers somewhere between 200 to 500 litai. OK, I thought, I have to evaluate everything on my own: if I were to help someone, how much would I want to get, and how much can I pay? The surgery lasts fifteen to twenty minutes, and Aida is young, and it's not life threatening."

"It didn't seem like a lot of money to me," Adomas continued. "I put 300 in the envelope, and my girlfriend bought this nice box of chocolates from a gourmet store. I wanted to add a little envelope with 100 litai for the nurse, but my girlfriend said it was too much, I shouldn't be raising prices," he laughed. The amount he settled on was 350. When Aida was admitted to the hospital, Adomas went into the surgeon's office to give him the envelope. "'Doctor, this is a thank you for you,' I told him. He said, 'No, no, there is no need,' and then I told him that the state doesn't pay the doctors enough. He took it. I gave the nurses a box of chocolates and told them to sweeten up their lives because they have a lot of work and need glucose."

I have heard numerous stories like this one, in which doctors who work at private clinics as consultants refer patients to public hospitals. In these cases, patients connect with doctors through private clinics and pay them legally for the initial consultation. The surgery is performed by the same doctors free of charge at the public hospital, and patients then thank the doctors with envelopes. Doctors and patients thus bypass both the owners of private clinics and the state. The enveloped practices function across the partial or semipublic and private realms.

In deciding how much to give the surgeon, Adomas seemed to be calculating quite rationally and following implicit rules. His assertion that the state does not pay doctors enough helped convince the doctor to accept the envelope and enabled both the doctor and Adomas to retain their dignity. The amount of money reflected his own assessment of how much he would want to receive, but it could not impose a financial burden on him, an engineer. Later he explained to me that of all people who were evading taxes, doctors were "the most deserving," because they "had no choice but to operate."

Yet Adomas perceived the enveloped care practices in another light, too. "Health is a delicate matter," he said. "When you need doctors, you think, OK, if I can afford it, I want to make sure that everything goes well. So, you have this natural desire to protect yourself from a hypothetical misfortune or failure, right? And what is the best tool to protect yourself from misfortunes?" While I was gathering my thoughts, Adomas answered his own question: "Insurance. This is a kind of insurance, too. When you go on a trip abroad, you buy travel insurance, which is optional, not necessary. But you do so hoping that nothing happens. It's like bribing God. I pay; I feel safer. It's the same with the doctors."

Adomas's attitude was a tangled mix of rational calculation and belief, inconsistent and mechanistic logic. For Adomas, as for many, the envelope represented more than a transaction between patient and doctor. He saw it as a bribe to God—a sacrifice that would help ensure quality care and a good outcome. At the same time, the money in the envelope, like the gift of chocolate, is a source of energy for those who work in hospitals. In effect, it preserves their vital functions, enabling good doctors to stay in Lithuania instead of moving to England, Ireland, or Norway. Adomas's case illustrates how mutual participation keeps the system together—not only in terms of Lithuania's particular culture of healing but the political economy of health care as well. While the envelope undoubtedly has symbolic efficacy for individual patients and perhaps for doctors, too, it has practical efficacy in keeping medical care available. It is debatable whether a single envelope has much effect, but as a whole, the practice of giving envelopes is crucial to keeping the health-care system working.

This chapter has begun to show how knowledge and beliefs about envelopes are transmitted and how they have a direct effect on the bodies of patients. When patients and their caregivers are caught in the envelope, they read all medical encounters through its lens. Adomas's very long bus ride back in the 1970s shows how this practice of caring and relating transcends political and economic shifts. Clinical practices and the will to care cannot be easily ascribed to socialist or neoliberal practices. In Lithuania, giving an envelope can relieve the anxiety of medical encounters, when patients and caregivers imagine the worst possible scenarios, as examples of Adomas, Brigita, Justinas, or Rasa show. At the same time all of them are ambivalent about giving. The act of giving is not limited to medical encounters; it extends through the dynamics of familial relations and caring collectives.

The envelope emerges as one of the key symbols that has the power to spur action, providing strategies for collapsing "complex experiences" and organizing action.[2] This symbol becomes an analytical tool and a practice for sorting out "complex and undifferentiated feelings and ideas" (Ortner 1973, 1340) about health, life, death, and survival. Envelopes provide Lithuanians with a way to conceptualize and share their experiences which, in turn, help perpetuate those practices. The envelope is a metaphor for social processes in health care and beyond. It is grounded in the social whole and affects how health-care experiences are articulated, lived, and enacted. That is how the envelope becomes meaningful and definitive for one's healing and the future. It gives people the power to face illness, provide care, and manage both unknown and definable social-economic-political constraints. At the same time, patients, caregivers, and doctors are being caught in the network of relations and put into positions not necessarily of their choosing. They all participate in sustaining enveloped care.

Interlude III

OF ENVELOPES AND GREEDY DOCTORS

Another canonical tale of doctors and envelopes differs from the chocolate box stories: rather than playing on the innocence or indifference of doctors who fail to notice gifts from patients, it mocks doctors who expect too much. I heard this story on a warm Friday afternoon in May 2010, at a traditional bathhouse on a lake, sitting with three friends who worked on regional development projects funded by the European Union. After we talked about the landscape and our different kinds of work, our conversation eventually turned to health and the honesty of doctors.

"This doctor R., an eye doctor in a nearby regional city, has no conscience (*sąžinės*); her appetite for envelopes is insatiable. She wants them on each visit, to the point that it is disgusting. And everybody knows about it. Well, she is a good doctor, but so dishonest. I hate dealing with her, but my father asks me to thank her every time I take him for a glaucoma check-up," sighed Renata.

"But there are some honest doctors left," her colleague Inga noted. "For instance, my sister-in-law took my niece to the surgeon for the second of two surgeries, and he didn't take the money the second time. He took just one envelope and told them that they had already thanked him. The honest ones know when to stop."

"You know what, I will tell you a story that my brother told me about this doctor that he heard about from a friend of his," offered Vilma, a music teacher in her forties.

> Here in this town or a neighboring one, there was a doctor. I think she was in charge of some commission, too. Anyway, she had a large appetite for gifts. She loved money. Everyone in the region knew about her, knew that she took bribes. This man, Antanas, or whatever his name was, needed documents, maybe to qualify for disability or something,

I don't exactly remember. He knew that without an envelope it would be impossible to get things done quickly. But he was smart. Listen to this: he put a fake one-hundred-dollar banknote in an envelope and gave it to her. The doctor took the money. When she wanted to spend it, she needed to exchange the dollars for litai. At the bank she found out that the money was fake. Of course, the bank called the police. She had to explain where she got the money. She had to have been ashamed! She couldn't possibly remember who gave her the envelope with the fake $100. Nice punishment, eh?

"I have heard this story!" Renata and Inga exclaimed almost in unison. I could have joined them because I also knew a version of the story. Then Inga said, "I will tell you another story, very similar to this one—except the envelope is empty." The other women started laughing and nodding, affirming their familiarity with this version of the story too. "It is a very similar story of a doctor who is shameless, always asking for money, you can't get anything from him without giving something. Once a patient who wanted to extend his disability benefits, knowing that the doctor wouldn't help without an envelope, gave him an empty one."

"I always feel better when I don't have to see the doctor's face when he is opening the envelope. I don't want to see the reaction—was that too little or too much?" Renata said to her nodding friends. Renata's commentary, incited by the reiteration of the tale, made her think about her own practices of giving envelopes to doctors.

In the different versions of this tale, the doctors are often specialists and members of commissions and committees that make decisions on disability and social welfare payments for the patients or primary caregivers. The protagonist of the story, who puts fake money in the envelope or gives an empty envelope to the doctor, is a patient or a primary caregiver for a parent, sibling, or spouse.

These tales reverse the power in the doctor-patient relationship. The patient, instead of having to satisfy the doctor's greed, gets what he needs without paying a bribe, and the doctor is punished. It seems that the intended result of the drama is shame or embarrassment, but the tale never has a clear ending. Does the doctor stop taking envelopes, curtail his/her appetite, or simply become warier and start checking envelopes immediately after getting them? This tale of punishment is also an expression of discontent and disempowerment.

In both versions of the story, whether the envelope contains fake money or is empty, the effect depends on the opacity of the envelope: the patient's ruse succeeds precisely because the envelope's contents are not visible. Justice is served within the realm of the envelope.

All these tales question the rationale for giving and taking envelopes and boxes. They also show the space of the subject. Both doctors and patients are part of the informal economy, linked with mechanics, bureaucrats, teachers, sales associates, and others. Patients, too, receive boxes and envelopes. By offering counterfeit money or an empty envelope, the patient enacts justice while bypassing state institutions. Both the doctor and the patient are involved in relationships of questionable legality: the patient has access to counterfeit money, and the doctor expects bribes.

The circulation of tales and of envelopes is interwoven; the former helps keep the latter alive. Doctors are generally cast as objects of sympathy. They are rarely faulted for accepting envelopes, except when they are perceived to be too greedy or too aggressive. These tales also convey respect for honest doctors and admit the inevitability of bad doctors. The practice is embedded in the social fabric; it is both opaque and transparent, with its own contradictions, justifications, and morals.

The practices associated with envelopes are "exercise an art of thinking," in Michel de Certeau's words (1984, 81). The tales include details of the way envelopes are given, how they are concealed, and their moral justifications; they weave a social fabric of care. They define the boundaries of the practice while invoking and negotiating local notions of honesty and justice. Certain behaviors are seen as exceeding the limits and are thus punishable. They open up concealed exchanges to discussions about their possibilities, advantages, miscommunications, humiliations, and limits. Although the concealed transactions might cause anxiety and disappointment, concealment allows both parties to evade scrutiny of the value of their offerings and services.

The tales also provoke discussions about the relations between care, objects, and people. They reveal a certain shared notion of care: concealed, uncertain, historically configured, and with its own innate logic. This is part of what I call enveloped care. Reiterations of these tales have therapeutic effects in that they help people to negotiate and cope with ambiguous practices and set the boundaries of acceptable practice.[1] The circulation and constant reconfiguration of these tales spur conceptual thinking about solving binaries and searching for compromises.

"I AM A DOCTOR"

Caught in Ambivalence

At the hospital in Vilnius, a doctor was accompanying a relative into a patient's room carrying a small, translucent orange bag in his hand. As he was passing by, Lina, a cardiologist, called out, "What is that small, girly bag for? Is it full of money? Don't give your money away!" The doctor replied, "It's better to give than to take."

During my fieldwork, doctors often underscored the complexity of the relationship between two modes of relating: giving and taking. They remembered how, as residents, they first encountered enveloped care. To those who grew up in doctors' families, offerings of food, favors, and money were already familiar. Some told me that at first, they were opposed to taking the envelopes, but then they ended up in situations where they felt they had to accept envelopes because it calmed their patients or because their senior colleagues advised them to do so. They told me stories of how a patient's condition deteriorated, or their relatives became upset when an envelope was refused.

Invariably, the Lithuanian doctors I talked with said that envelopes did not affect their medical decisions. They identified strongly with the idealized role of the doctor and claimed to act solely in the interest of the patient's well-being. Doctors were often conflicted about the practices around envelopes. Those I spent more time with distinguished between patients who gave them gifts out of gratitude and those who gave gifts insincerely. They tried to avoid the latter but did not always succeed. At the same time, doctors viewed gift offerings as a sign of achievement and were proud of being recognized as worthy of receiving envelopes.

This chapter explores how doctors negotiate ethical issues, the practice of medicine, and the political economy through relations of care that envelopes signify. Doctors deal with the dilemmas of enveloped care at every stage of their profession. Young resistant doctors I observed would ultimately give in to the system of envelopes, which involved learning to cultivate the ambiguous position of not asking for envelopes but being grateful when they were given. They faced dilemmas of whether to take these envelopes, how not to show that they wanted them, and how not to be seen as a briber but rather as honest and good. Receiving envelopes signified a measure of respect and recognition from their patients and, perhaps, their colleagues. Moreover, most of the doctors had been on the other side of such transactions. They had family members who asked them to settle accounts with other doctors, and they, too, had given envelopes and used their connections to see the best doctors. They often felt caught between the two modes of relating: giving and taking, entangled between responsibilities as doctors and their obligations as neighbors, relatives, friends, or colleagues.

Doctors' practices of giving, receiving, and conceptualizing envelopes illustrate how they draw the lines between bribes, gifts, and payments. Some doctors view envelopes and the commodification of care as challenges to medical authority. However, others consider the practice of enveloped care as interfering less with good doctoring, and hence more ethical than selling health at private clinics. Doctors' portrayals of their working conditions and the constraints that new regulations place on their roles in the medical field nuance our understanding of shifting economies of health in postsocialist Lithuania. Their stories and perspectives reveal how envelopes constitute relations between doctors and patients, while they also play a role in defining the relations between the health-care sector and the state. The previous chapter showed how patients invest hope in the envelope and feel empowered to face medical encounters. This chapter explores how doctors are caught in the ambiguity that envelopes embody. Envelopes destabilize doctors and challenge their authority while also recognizing them for being good doctors.

Becoming a Doctor

"So what! Chill out. Get used to it. It has happened to me too," said a third-year resident, Aida, to a new resident, Kornelija. The latter was still blushing after a patient, a man in his late sixties, had hugged her from behind, kissed her on the cheek, and said, "Thank you, my doctor, I am leaving now," as he slipped a banknote (50 or 100 litai, judging from the color) into her pocket.

I witnessed this scene in the residents' office. The patient had spent five days in the cardiology unit receiving treatment for a heart arrhythmia. Before leaving the unit, he stopped by the office to say goodbye to Kornelija. As he embraced her, she instantly turned red and protested in a shaky voice, "No! No! What are you doing?" (*Nereikia! Ka jus darote? Tikrai nereikia!*). "It's OK. I want to thank you," said the man. He waved, wishing all of us good luck, and left. The residents exchanged glances. Kornelija was speechless and looked horrified by the envelope and the unwanted physical contact.

Aida and two other residents tried to calm Kornelija down, telling her she would get used to encounters with patients in which she would have to decide whether to accept or refuse their gifts and how to manage relationships with patients. Becoming a doctor in Lithuania involves not only learning to read charts, make diagnoses, monitor medications, and fill out paperwork but also dealing with envelopes. Kornelija was aware of the envelopes circulating in the clinics in Lithuania. She had seen envelopes being offered to her senior colleagues and fellow residents, but this patient's gesture caught her by surprise and embarrassed her. Several weeks later, I saw an envelope sticking out of Kornelija's pocket as she returned from a meeting with a patient's son. She did not blush. She was smiling.

When I talked with Aida about the incident, she expressed similarly conflicted feelings about the envelopes. "We are not asking [for money], are we? You saw it." Her "are we?" seemed to express uncertainly and request reassurance. Aida was admired by patients and medical staff alike. She had wit and personality. She loved patients and, more often than other doctors, came back from her rounds with bars of chocolate, boxes of coffee, and other sweets, which she enjoyed. Yet gifts of money seemed to make her uncomfortable. "It is very unpleasant to me," she sighed, sitting on the sofa in the residents' office. "The other day there was this old woman who looked like my grandmother. She slipped 20 litai into my pocket. At that moment, I thought maybe she didn't have money, but she was still giving me something. I was thinking about my grandma. I felt sad. So I gave the money back, telling her, 'Grandma, please get something nice for yourself, I don't need this.'" But the old woman refused to take the money. She pushed it back to Aida, who tried again to give it back. In the end, Aida said, "Grandma got upset and forced the money on me. I gave up."

At the beginning of her residency, Aida had also resisted accepting an envelope from an older woman, but a nurse advised her not to be arrogant and to accept the money. According to the nurse, the patient would be happier if Aida accepted the money; otherwise, the old woman might think that she was giving it in the wrong way or not giving enough. Over time, Aida had developed her own code of conduct for these situations. She felt it was inappropriate to accept an envelope before the patient left the clinic. At that point, she said, "You feel that you have done something good. But when you accept an envelope before care is provided, you feel terrible. What if the patient doesn't get better? Once you accept the envelope, patients start commanding you, telling you what tests and drugs they want, how long they want to stay, where they want to be sent for rehabilitation. But you can't do everything they want, especially if you don't think they need these additional tests."

In Aida's view, patients use envelopes to alter the power balance of the doctor-patient relationship. Patients and their relatives want care that meets their own understanding of their needs, sometimes expecting doctors to depart from the treatment protocols defined by the State Insurance Fund and the hospital administration. I see this situation as somewhat similar to the practices in Soviet health care described by Michelle Rivkin-Fish (2005), in which patients seek personalized relationships with doctors to counter bureaucratic power and indifference. Lithuanian patients are challenging not only bureaucratic constraints but also the doctor's medical authority by demanding certain tests or procedures. This goes beyond cultivating a friendly relationship with the doctor. Aida perceived these gestures as a challenge to her medical knowledge and authority. For the time being, she said, she managed to avoid accepting envelopes before the patients' discharge by telling them that first she must talk to her senior colleague. "It works while I am a resident," she said, but later on, she would have "more power and authority to refuse or accept." She also spoke of the financial and political implications of accepting envelopes. "Our salaries are not that high, so it turns out that patients are paying us." But this, in turn, creates an argument for not raising doctors' salaries, because "everybody knows that we get thank-yous." Aida, like many young doctors, felt caught in the ambivalence of the envelope. Her comments express shame, sadness, gratitude, and dependency, as well as a sense of professional authority. These conflicted feelings are a part of becoming and being a doctor in Lithuania. Aida is trying to be a conscientious doctor and to set her boundaries. She accepts an experienced nurse's advice to not be arrogant by refusing a patient's envelope because arrogance runs contrary to being the good doctor she aspires to become. At the same time, giving in and accepting envelopes makes her complicit in a practice she once despised. Neither she nor Kornelija imagined they would be doctors who take envelopes. Moreover, Aida worries that accepting envelopes undermines the professional authority of doctors by making them dependent on patients. For young doctors this is a particularly sensitive issue because patients often mistrust them and question their decisions. Indeed, more than one patient told me, "If you don't give an envelope, some resident will practice on your body."

By contrast, a young surgeon, Lukas, told me that he was not ashamed that patients wanted to thank him. Lukas was a top student who had spent a few semesters abroad through the Socrates program (an EU student exchange program) and hoped to stay at Vilnius Hospital and pursue an academic career. He grew up in Telšiai, a provincial town, where his mother was a municipal accountant, and his father worked as a truck driver for an international logistics company. Like Aida, Lukas emphasized that he never asked patients for money. He vividly remembered the first time he received an envelope. It was one of the first supervised surgeries where he had a real chance to operate. An envelope was, he said, the last thing on his mind. Rather, Lukas was worried about the patient, an older man. He went to check on him perhaps more frequently than usual. The man's daughter put an envelope into his pocket a day before the patient's discharge. "I didn't expect that. I felt grateful," Lukas said. I asked him whether he felt he deserved the envelope. "Now I think I did, but not then." I asked him if, perhaps, someone could have understood his unusually frequent visits as provocations or tacit requests for an envelope. Lukas looked at me with disbelief and said, "Perhaps one could see it this way, I guess, . . . but I sincerely cared."

Lukas gets envelopes once in a while but fewer than his senior colleagues. The money supplements his resident stipend and salary, preventing him from having to ask his parents for money or take out loans. Lukas and his girlfriend, also a student, are renting a studio apartment in Vilnius. They drive a beat-up, fifteen-year-old Volkswagen Golf that needs constant repairs. "That car gets all my envelopes," he joked.

Talking cautiously, weighing every word, Lukas described envelopes as a symbol of patients' gratitude and a reward for being a good and caring doctor, reiterating how patients valued doctors based on their individual experiences— affective (bio)metrics. He was not asking for envelopes but was grateful to receive them. They made him feel appreciated but also deserving. It will take years for Lukas to overcome patients' fears of young doctors and become recognized as a good doctor, which saddened him because, as he put it, he and other young doctors tried harder and were supervised by the best doctors. Kornelija, Aida, and Lukas were quickly caught up in existing affective practices and modes of doctoring that go beyond the biomedical. This included negotiating envelopes, professional ethics, and material constraints.

The struggle to align biomedical competence and affective side of medical care is not unique to Lithuanian medical residents; it is one of the core issues embedded in medical training. Rachel Prentice, in her ethnography of anatomy and surgery education in the United States, notes that physicians develop "unique regimes of practice, culturally distinct styles of interacting with persons, bodies, and pathologies" (2013, 9). Byron Good and Mary Jo DelVecchio

Good (1993) examine the tensions between competence and caring in American medical training, showing how medical knowledge is constructed in the intuited relationship between biomedicine and the social organization of medicine (see also Good 1994). Lithuanian patients complained that even if doctors were competent, often they were "cold" and lacked any bedside manner, and thus perceived them as uncaring. Doctors must simultaneously learn to see patients' bodies as objects of knowledge and embody caring qualities. Good and DelVecchio Good define this caring as "a language of relationships, of attitudes and emotions, and of innate qualities of persons" (1993, 93). This caring is just as important as sophisticated biomedical knowledge in creating a constructive and satisfying doctor-patient relationship (DelVecchio Good, Munakata, Kobayashi, Mattingly, Good 1994, 858). As Cheryl Mattingly (2010) notes, caring doctors foster friendly connections and go beyond "mere professionalism." Going beyond professionalism for medical residents like Kornelija, Lukas, or Aida is becoming an intricate part of enveloped care. They work in conditions where patients interpret medical encounters through the lens of the envelope. A lack of warmth was frequently understood as a provocation and a signal to give an envelope. Alternatively, showing care also resulted in envelopes. Lithuanian doctors must navigate the relationship between competence and care in the context of these informal practices, whereas medical practitioners in the United States must deal with those issues in the context of the formal market-oriented health-insurance industry.

The anthropological study of the role of gifts and money in clinical practice has been largely restricted to postsocialist contexts (Bazylevych 2009, 2010; Brotherton 2012; Rivkin-Fish 2005; Salmi 2003; Stan 2012). The topic has received attention in professional medical journals (Drew, Stoeckle, and Billings 1983; Lycklom 1998) and has been discussed in the context of mental health (Ootes, Pols, Tonkens, and Willems 2013) and nursing homes (Buch 2014). These authors note that while gift-giving is officially frowned on and largely hidden from view, it nonetheless occurs commonly enough in everyday medical practice in the United States and Great Britain. Gifts break everyday routines, address imbalances in doctor-patient relations, and have a sacrificial element (Drew et al. 1983, 399–402). They personalize managed care (Lycklom 1998) and show that caring is not only a technical, medical procedure but a social activity, as well (Ootes et al. 2013). Vincanne Adams (1998) studied doctoring in Nepal and described how doctors negotiated gifts. She noted that Nepalese doctors were troubled when accepting gifts from patients before treatment because it reinforced nonmodern beliefs about making offerings to gods and entrusted unrealistic powers to the biomedical field. As we saw in the previous chapter, Lithuanian patients also granted powers to their doctors, but they were inseparable from the material power of the envelopes to conjure up the best kinds of relationships, to ensure better care, and to prove relatives were caring.

"I am not asking"—words reiterated in almost all of my conversations with residents—sounded like a mantra, an embodied practice of interacting with patients. Yet the presence of an envelope inevitably frames interpretations of the medical encounter. Envelopes disrupt the routines of patient care. They smooth the doctor-patient relationship while at the same time casting suspicion on it. The envelope is a direct and indirect actor in doctor-patient encounters. While Lithuanian doctors did not worry much about their patients' superstitious beliefs or attributions of almost godlike powers to them, they were troubled by the power that the envelopes could exert. They saw accepting envelopes before treatment as constraining their professionalism and possible treatment options. Knowing how and when to accept or gracefully decline offers of envelopes is an essential, learned skill for Lithuanian doctors. Furthermore, the ambivalent position of not asking has become the mark of the good and caring doctor.

Those "Other" Doctors

All the doctors and patients I interviewed claimed to know examples of the other kind of doctors (*kiti gydytojai*)—the ones who spun time, explicitly asked for money or gifts, or differentiated among patients based on how much was in the envelopes. Such doctors were considered greedy, unprofessional, and unethical. They thought about money, not patients; they were slow at adjusting medications for patients; and most important, they appeared disengaged. According to patients, these doctors were not friendly and did the bare minimum, complaining about their low salaries while wearing Rolex watches. They felt entitled to envelopes. Their white coats had oversized pockets; they were masters at extorting envelopes. When they accepted the envelopes, they did so with condescension and without a sign of gratitude or appreciation. Patients and doctors often referred to these "other" doctors as Soviet. When I asked what the adjective meant in this context, I was told that it stood for rude and abrupt, grumpy, a butcher. Such doctors made you feel uncomfortable asking questions and did not listen. Only envelopes could animate their grim faces and elicit smiles and invitations to patients to please come back again. One would expect that twenty years after Soviet rule ended, this adjective would be attributed to the generation of doctors who had practiced medicine since Soviet socialism, but Soviet was not only a generational category. It referred to the lack of sensible communication and commitment within medical institutional settings. In this sense, the envelope is a complex negotiation over the provision and definition of good medical care and who defines it.

Doctors differentiated themselves from these other doctors by a variety of means, including medical specialty. Surgeons thought that internists, cardiologists, and psychiatrists more often became these other doctors. Young doctors were critical of senior colleagues. Among the patients I spoke to, few claimed to have had personal contact with this kind of doctor, though everyone seemed to have a secondhand story about them. At a dinner party, I heard Daiva, a preschool teacher, vividly retelling a story about one of the other doctors from a friend. Since the story was recent, Daiva introduced me to Jolita, who shared her experience of the other doctor.

Jolita, a thirty-seven-year-old teacher from a regional town, encountered this in Dr. K., a well-known surgeon and professor of medicine who occasionally published health advice articles in glossy weekly magazines. Jolita was suspicious of a mole on her hand and went to a private clinic in Vilnius for tests. The mole was found to be malignant, and Jolita was advised to have it removed promptly. The doctor at the clinic arranged for her to have the surgery at the university hospital within two days.

Jolita asked her friends about the appropriate amount to put in the envelope for the surgeon. She was told not to worry because the surgery was minor, even though it was very important. It's not your heart or stomach, her friends told her, and she agreed. Jolita went to the hospital's outpatient surgery center and had the surgery done by Dr. K. There were no complications. After the surgery, Jolita was surprised that the surgeon started asking her various questions: "Where do you live? What do you do?" "I was answering these questions and waiting for the moment to give the envelope with 200 litai in it to the surgeon; the man treated me fast, I felt I needed to be grateful. And then I realized that he knew the answers to these questions. He was simply waiting for the money," remembered Jolita. She finished dressing and approached the surgeon to give him the money. But what happened was highly unexpected. The doctor took a small piece of paper and wrote a number on it: 800. "I looked at him and at the number. I was shocked and humiliated. I said to him, 'Doctor, I have only 200 litai,' and I put the money on the table. He didn't even look at me. I felt dizzy. I was disgusted and left as soon as I could. Shameless. Can you imagine, Rima? Briber! And he calls himself a doctor!" Jolita called the surgeon a briber not because he took the money but because he broke the unwritten rules of the exchange by specifying an amount. Also, with his superfluous questions, he was provoking Jolita to give. His actions prevented her from feeling grateful and reframed the doctor-patient relationship as one of bribery.

Donata, a first-year resident, told me that she was "afraid of doctors who lost their humanity (*žmogiškumą*), those who work only for envelopes. I hope I won't be like them. I will not follow the principle that if palms are not greased, the system doesn't work. I will not allow myself to be bought." Losing humanity for Daiva and other young doctors meant the lack of empathy and crossing the boundary from not asking to extortions of envelopes, like in the case of Jolita. When I asked Donata whether she would accept envelopes from the patients who wanted to thank her, she said, "Yes, I will accept gratitude, a gratuity." In her strong condemnation of other doctors, Donata distinguished between sincere giving and taking and a mercenary attitude. Humanity for her was based on sincerity, gratitude, and compassion, in contrast to the mercantile logic of the market and/or the protocols of the hospital and the state. A "human" doctor, according to her, is compassionate as well as caring, does not put money first, and sees patients as human beings. This kind of doctor also accepts envelopes as signs of gratitude and recognition.

Patients, caretakers, and doctors drew their subtle lines between what was ethically acceptable and what was not, who was good and who was not. As these stories illustrate, tales about other doctors circulated, giving them the reputation of accepting bribes. It was not the presence of the envelope with money in the medical encounters that people condemned, but the way it came about in the encounter. The distinction between good doctors and other doctors is fluid and contingent. At times, depending on their workload, many good doctors might cross the line. When the implicit rules of the relationship are not respected, then the doctor, according to the patient, becomes the other kind of doctor, and the envelope is transformed from a mark of appreciation into a bribe or illegal payment. As Rivkin-Fish observes, "Subtle distinctions in the way the objects were presented became signifiers for the kind of exchange being conducted" (2005,168). Indeed, the manner and mode of offering and accepting money are crucial in determining the nature of the exchange and its relational modes.

Accepting Ambivalence

One morning I walked into Marija's office and saw a red gift bag on the floor next to her desk. An energetic woman in her late thirties, Marija was one of my key informants, someone I had talked with for more than three years and had shadowed several times. She caught me staring at the gift bag. "Yesterday a patient left that bag. I wanted to give it to my nurses, but I looked inside, and next to the bottle of brandy and chocolates there was an envelope," said Marija. "There have been times when I didn't even notice; I didn't know who gave it to me or when. Once I found an envelope in the files."

Some of Marija's patients, according to her, were slipping money into her pockets or among the files on her desk or leaving them inside gift bags, chocolate boxes, and books. Some accompanied the money with notes saying, "Thank you, doctor, for helping me. Please buy yourself or your kids something you like—perfume or wine you love. I didn't know what to give you."

"How much do you get in these envelopes?" I asked her.

"Anywhere between 10 and 400 hundred litai," she said.

"Four hundred litai? Why?" I asked, knowing that she did not do surgeries and most of her patients were not rich.

"You think I am not worth 400?" Marija laughed.

"Who gave it to you?" I continued.

"There is a man, a patient of mine, who comes back to me every year and gives the same amount each time. He has a good job. Money is not an issue for him—but seriously, I don't know why."

"Everyone thinks that the doctor is doing you a huge favor, but it is our job, and we do it every day," she added. "If you invite patients to come back soon for whatever reason and listen to them, they think you are doing it for the money. Some doctors do that. For instance, this doctor R.—we all know he pays too much attention to money. He drops hints for the patients. It is so obvious and not acceptable. It shouldn't be that way." Marija was reinforcing that it was permissible to accept envelopes as long as you do not ask for them and condemning the other doctor who provoked patients.

Marija and other doctors differentiated envelopes not by the amount but by the intentions behind them: whether the envelope was given as a sincere thank-you gift for the doctor's care, or whether its purpose was to buy the doctor and influence the treatment process. "When the patients want to give me money upfront, when they demand things—giving an envelope and making their intentions explicit—for example, [to obtain] a disability pension or sick leave, something I don't think I can do—I don't accept this way of buying me."

According to Marija, in such cases a simple "No, no, thank you" leads patients to think that they are giving too little. "I have to fight with them—use stronger words," she explained. However, when Marija thought that accepting an envelope would calm the patient or the relative without indicating a willingness to compromise her professional judgment, she did so. In this case, she considered the envelope as an expression of trust in her as a doctor.

Marija, like other doctors, received the money in widely varying amounts. Some months, the envelopes almost amounted to a second salary; other months, she received only one or two. The most generous givers were returned Lithuanian migrants who accompanied their relatives and gave on their behalf. "People who lived in England, Norway, or Ireland appreciate us more. They went to the doctors there and were not attended carefully, not listened to, given paracetamol, and released. So they come back home for treatment." These patients were less demanding and more appreciative.

Occasionally patients and their relatives came to talk to her and made implied promises at the beginning of treatment. For instance, according to Marija, they would say, "'Doctor, please help us—switch the schedule around, make calls to other doctors, or something. We will not be in debt, we will thank you later, we will be very grateful,' and they leave without saying goodbye or thank you. You think that you are doing a good job, but you never know how people see it." Such promises might not materialize into an envelope.

Marija emphasized that she did not rely on the income from envelopes to plan her budget. "You can't count on them—they vary month by month, depending on the patients. I don't rely on them. I am grateful to the patients." When the 2008 financial crisis hit and austerity measures were implemented in Lithuania, she said, patients' salaries shrank, and they started giving less. She noted, "Pharmaceutical companies are a guaranteed source of income; envelopes are not. For giving one lecture or participating in a clinical trial I get much more, but that's not the point. I am a doctor."

Compared to general physicians and other specialists, surgeons seemed to enjoy a more stable income from envelopes. People took invasive techniques like surgeries seriously, I was told, and were much more generous. Sometimes, surgeons' refusals to accept envelopes were perceived as signs of a poor prognosis. Patients and their relatives sought out surgeons with good reputations, using all kinds of social connections, including envelopes, in the hope of getting treatment from those they understood to be the best. Vilnius Hospital and the surgery unit where I conducted my research were perceived to be among the very best institutions with the best doctors.

Vidas, who is in his late thirties, is a surgeon who has been operating for twelve years and performs 150 surgeries a year. With his messy hair and distracted look, he reminded me more of a philosopher than a surgeon. Vidas was the least productive surgeon in his unit, at least as measured by the envelopes he received. Few patients gave Vidas envelopes asking him to operate on them. Compared to his colleagues, Vidas had more urgent patients who did not give anything. "Sometimes I have only three or four patients, while others have double that. I don't make an effort to get more. Patients don't often ask me to be their surgeon. I am not that doctor yet, even though my cemetery is very small." Though Vidas graduated at the top of his class and was respected by his colleagues, patients did not recognize his skill. This may have been partly because many of his patients came from the emergency room and needed immediate surgery.

Although Vidas said he felt rewarded by patients' gratitude, he still felt uneasy about envelopes when he received them: "When I get money, I feel that I am expected to do more than I can. It's not easy. Patients think that if they pay, you will make them healthy. There is too much responsibility. I need to get a thicker skin." The surgeon linked his youth to what he defined as his uneasiness in receiving envelopes. But he also saw receiving envelopes as recognition for being a good doctor. For Vidas, as for the Ukrainian doctors Maryna Bazylevych (2010a, 2010b) studied, informal payments are a source of social capital and prestige.

Furthermore, taking an envelope made Vidas feel obliged "to sit and talk with the patient, listen to their life stories," even though he had "a ton of things to do." These obligatory chitchats with patients often destabilized him as a surgeon, he said. He would rather use this time to prepare for surgery. At the same time, he acknowledged that envelopes mattered to him. If it were not for the envelopes, he would have moved to Britain by now for work. Other doctors also told me that if they did not have the supplementary income from envelopes, they would have to seriously consider working abroad. According to some studies, since 2004, somewhere between 4 and 8 percent of Lithuanian doctors (mostly anesthesiologists, radiologists, and optometrists) have moved to Britain and Scandinavia; these are mostly young doctors who had not developed relationships (*pririšti*) with their patients (Taljūnaite 2012). Vidas was reliant on the system of envelopes, even though it made him question his doctoring abilities.

Vidas's colleague Marius, a successful surgeon in his fifties, operates on 280 to 300 patients a year. When I was at the hospital, patients came directly to him almost every day, with and without referrals, asking him to operate on them, even though for nonemergency surgery his long waitlist meant deferring a procedure for a month or more. He was outgoing and witty, constantly making jokes bordering on black humor, sexism, and rudeness. But nurses adored him; if a patient asked them which surgeon to choose, they very often suggested Marius. On the website that ranks Lithuanian doctors and health-care facilities, comments on his profile called him "an angel in a white coat."[1] At the time, the website also included information about the frequency and amount of gifts each doctor had received. About 50 percent of patients gave gifts to Marius in the range of 100–300 litai. At the same time, many patients criticized his rudeness and arrogance.

Marius told me his view of gifts and envelopes: "By no means should a doctor ask for or somehow hint at a gift. If a doctor indicates that he or she desires money and asks a patient for it, then it is a bribe. But if a patient knocks on my door and simply asks particularly for me to operate and then gives me a little envelope for that—it is a gift. Our people want particular doctors; they want a relationship. In the West you choose a clinic, not a surgeon." Marius emphasized that a doctor's personality and ability to affectively connect with patients mattered as much or even more than biomedical competence. When I asked him what he did about patients who did not offer envelopes, he replied sarcastically, "Oh yes, we keep them stacked on a rack waiting to die. What do you think I do? I operate. I am a doctor." Marius perceived envelopes from the patients as signs of recognition and rewards for his excellent practice. He radiated an almost godlike sense of authority and entitlement. Even though Vidas refused to accept envelopes before surgeries and seemed overall more accessible to his patients, I noted on a few occasions that patients assigned to Vidas asked to be reassigned to Marius.

These three doctors perceived envelopes as gratitude for their good doctoring. Even though Vidas considered envelopes to be destabilizing, their absence made him doubt his abilities. Their experiences illustrate how patients did not reward doctors equally or logically, but rather based on patients' affective (bio)metrics—their experience of being cared for. General practitioner Marija could not rely on envelopes to plan her budget, while that was not the case for Marius, the surgeon. Doctors seemed caught in the practices of envelopes that they perceived both as rewarding and unsettling. None of them had clear ideas for how to break this cycle. Doctors wanted bigger salaries but also doubted that this would stop these enveloped practices. Some envisioned private clinics as an alternative, but others were skeptical.

Helping, Not Selling

Loreta, a family doctor in her forties, first worked for a private clinic and then switched back to the public polyclinic. She compared her work at both institutions and the different practices and attitudes toward money that prevailed at each by contrasting selling health care with receiving envelopes. Loreta interpreted envelopes as a sign of gratitude and "an expression of patients' love for themselves," directly relating envelopes to the will to care. According to her, the act of giving made patients and their families feel better. With a touch of irony, she noted, "Patients love themselves more when they need surgery," meaning that surgeons and specialists received more and larger envelopes than family doctors did.

Loreta's patients brought her gifts such as chocolate, flowers, and fruit from their gardens, handmade slippers, and money. "If I ate all the chocolate I get, I don't know what would happen to me," she laughed. Older women often gave 10 litai in an envelope and were pushy, she said, "They are afraid that I may not treat them well. But I treat all my patients equally. And they get upset if I don't want to take it." Those who gave her money often told her to buy something for herself. She was particularly touched by an older patient who brought children's books, knowing from the photos on her desk that she had a little boy. Loreta spoke with great sympathy about this old woman, describing her gifts as coming from the heart. It seemed that Loreta valued sincere relationships with her patients as much as they did. She appreciated being perceived not only as a caring doctor but as the mother of a small boy.

I was intrigued by how she dealt with the patients who used envelopes to get state-subsidized sick leave (ranging from three days to two months), which required a doctor's authorization.[2] Some patients did not meet the criteria for paid sick leave, but she granted it anyway. Loreta explained, "They could work— they had a runny nose but no fever—so formally they can't get this leave. But I allow myself to think that maybe the patient indeed feels bad, doesn't want to go to work, doesn't feel like working, even though they don't have a fever, only a sore throat. People are overworked these days." She added that she does not tolerate patients who request paid sick leave too often. In such cases, she always recommends that they make an appointment with a psychiatrist or psychologist at the same polyclinic.

During my fieldwork, I met patients who begged their family doctors for sick leave authorizations with 50 litai in an envelope and a convincing story. For some, it offered protection from losing their jobs when austerity measures were implemented in the aftermath of the 2008 financial crisis, and it was illegal to lay off employees who were on sick leave. Going on sick leave allowed them to look for another job or fortify themselves for the changes ahead. Some middle-class patients took sick leave because their employers offered little or no paid vacation.

Sick leave, it is important to note, is not a postsocialist phenomenon. It was also a tactic that patients and doctors used to cope with the economy of shortages during socialism. Under conditions of a compulsory work regime, people, in particular those who participated in the informal economy, used sick leave to develop their private enterprises, while others used that time to stand in lines, work on their private collective gardens, or vacation. Thus, obtaining sick leave via envelopes has been one way to employ biology as a resource, whether to stay afloat in the case of the diminishing welfare state or escape the limitations of state socialism.

Anthropologists discussed how biomedicine and one's biology could become one of the few avenues to access social benefits that otherwise would not be available (Fassin 2009; Petryna 2002; Ticktin 2006). In certain contexts, for instance for immigrant populations, diagnosis can pave a path to citizenship.)[3] Such sick leave cases in socialist and postsocialist contexts differ from and are similar to the interpretations of biological citizenship.[4] They mark one of the strains of biological citizenship. Sick leave tactics, facilitated by the informal economy, are connected to configurations of political regimes, their systems of social welfare, and their faults. They also emphasize the role of medicine and the rights, privileges, and entitlements attached to them. They illustrate the sociality of medicine; that is, how the social employs medicine and sick roles, manipulates its commodification, and acts as a compensatory mechanism to obtain welfare. Sick leave manipulations worked to protect or expand social livelihoods. The ways sick leave was employed to counteract the lack of opportunities for legal self-expression illustrated the cracks in state socialism.

Then, during socialism, and now, amid capitalism, envelopes facilitated using biology as a resource to enhance well-being. They continue to work as a tactic, a temporary shelter or relief, prepaid parallel insurance to enhance livelihoods under late capitalism. These tactics are also expressions of the will to care. In contemporary Lithuania, informal transactions help to sustain participation in the formal labor market and class belonging, even if only for a short period of time. They safeguard against the pitfalls of the welfare state as well as manipulate the gaps in the state and the market. In his study of Cuban medicine, Sean Brotherton (2012) shows how mutual solidarity between doctors and patients fills the gaps left by the state. He describes cases, also in the context of informal exchanges, when doctors selectively report certain cases of disease to the state and thus abstain from the surveillance of patients. In a similar vein, Doctor Loreta sees herself as helping people to mitigate the shortfalls of the economic, political, social systems. By helping others, she helps them sustain their own lives.

Despite her willingness to accept envelopes, however, Loreta told me she did not want to "sell health as a product." After working at a private clinic as a family doctor for a few years, she quit and switched to the public polyclinic, even though it meant seeing twenty-five patients a day instead of ten and dealing with all the problems of an underfunded, state-run facility, such as crashing computer systems and piles of paperwork. At the private clinic, according to Loreta, management and business matters were interfering with her role as a doctor: "I was reminded multiple times to refer patients to other doctors and do more tests, to generate more income. I hated that. At times it felt that I was working at a store selling health, but I am a doctor, not a salesperson. The diagnosis, tests, and treatment plan are for me to decide."

The young, middle-class patients Loreta saw at the private clinic usually were not seriously ill but simply busy people who did not want to wait in line at the polyclinic. "Patients would come with a sore throat, and I was urged to order multiple tests—a full-body ultrasound, a full blood panel. But these patients were mostly young and did not have chronic illnesses. Nonsense. They simply wanted to see the doctor the same day," said Loreta. Sometimes, according to her, patients simply needed to rest, drink raspberry or linden flower tea, and talk. She found it troubling to make her patients spend hundreds or thousands of litai for unnecessary tests and treatments.

For Loreta, taking envelopes from patients at the polyclinic was more ethically acceptable than ordering needless tests and prescriptions at the private clinic. (Official salaries at both places are very similar.) She saw public and private health care as parallel ethical regimes with different sets of values. By shifting from one regime to another, she was engaging in consideration of meanings and values attached to what Didier Fassin calls "life as such"—life shaped by political choices, the moral economies of contemporary societies, and concrete ways in which individual groups are treated "under which principles and in the name of which morals, implying which inequalities and misrecognitions" (Fassin 2009, 57). Loreta's attitude toward envelopes and her handling of the sick leave cases emphasized the biographical rather than the biological aspects of patient care. Her choices highlight the dilemma of the transformation from informal payments to copayments and the problems of health commodification through privatization. Should health care be governed by principles of formal justice and transparency, efficiency and rationality, or by patients' well-being?

New Economics, New Limits

The practice of giving and taking envelopes is often ascribed to the low salaries and shortage economy that prevailed under socialism and the economic turbulence associated with the transition to capitalism: a lack of medications, supplies, and technologies, as well as isolation from the global medical community.[5] Lithuanian doctors' salaries lag behind the incomes of medical practitioners in Western Europe as well as the salaries of top managers and IT professionals in Lithuania. However, the link between envelopes and low salaries is not straightforward. Although doctors' salaries more than doubled between 2004 and 2008, the enveloped practices did not decrease. Neither patients nor doctors expressed a belief that paying medical practitioners significantly higher salaries would immediately eliminate the circulation of envelopes. Doctors often brought up their inadequate salaries in our conversations. But they also emphasized that low pay did not prevent them from being competent and caring doctors.

After more than twenty years of capitalism, the notion of the shortage economy has acquired a new meaning. It no longer refers to a shortage of supplies, crumbling infrastructure, or limited access to technologies and medications. In the twenty-first century, doctoring encounters other types of constraints, such as a shortage of time, a cumbersome bureaucracy, and rigid protocols. The doctors I spoke with did not blame the system, as some medical practitioners in post-Soviet Russia and Ukraine did (Bazylevych 2014; Rivkin-Fish 2005), but rather talked about quotas and financial allocations, the growing care needs of an aging population, market solutions, and management standards.

Doctors who practiced during the Soviet period emphasized the progress of biomedicine since that time. "I started working in this hospital in 1982. It's like night and day if I compare my cases, [in terms of] death rates and treatment options," noted Regina, a cardiologist in her late fifties. "You must know that cardiac care in Lithuania was among the best in the Soviet Union; people would come seeking help even from Leningrad. But I am telling you: night and day."[6] She told me that she was a bit envious of the opportunities now available to young doctors, such as the possibility of studying abroad and doing important research.

Although Regina certainly was not nostalgic for the socialist era, she was disappointed by the increasing bureaucracy of the current system: "Soviet bureaucracy was a piece of cake (*smulkmena*) compared to the EU." Nowadays, she said, everything had to be documented, and every case might be scrutinized. She was exasperated by the protocols of accountability and the possibility of being sued by patients or their relatives. "People were dying before the 1990s, and nobody made a big deal out of it. Now, if your patient dies or blames you for complications, you go through investigations, or, even worse, you can end up in court." She pointed out that despite technological advances, medicine still had limits. This conversation happened when Regina was filing paperwork on a deceased patient.

Regina, like other doctors, lamented the ways new protocols restricted a doctor's autonomy. She expressed concern with regulations limiting hospitalization days and procedures according to protocols for different diseases. "I have to do what the rules prescribe, and not what I think is best. I cannot keep a patient and carefully observe him or her for a month. In that sense, as a doctor, I have less freedom," she said. Doctors "knew better" because they were professionals and experts. She was critical of both the old and new obstacles to her idea of good doctoring. Nowadays, medicine is more like management than a caring profession.

The younger doctors knew about health care during socialism only through the stories of their parents and older colleagues. Doctors took pride in being connected to the global medical community through attending conferences (funded by pharmaceutical companies), participating in medical research, and working with new technologies and drugs. At Vilnius Hospital, many doctors participated in medical research and worked for companies that conducted clinical trials.[7] Even so, doctors felt their pay was low. Some had second jobs in polyclinics and worked as consultants for private clinics. "In the news, they say that Lithuania spends a lot of money on health care, so people think we earn millions," Regina said. "But the money goes to buying equipment and subsidizing expensive drugs, so you can imagine how much money that is." Unfortunately, according to her, doctors and residents are not paid enough, so "patients are supporting us. It is hard to imagine how the cycle will break."

General practitioners and specialists alike complained about the number of patients that they had to see and the ever-increasing amount of paperwork. "We are working under conditions of a chronic shortage of time," said Rasa, a family doctor. Their paperwork involved filling out forms for the hospital, Social Services (Sodra), and the State Health Insurance Fund, as well as making sure the files were complete and accurate in case a patient filed a complaint that would lead to a state audit. Every time I saw Rasa, she was annoyed by electronic systems that crashed and forced her to duplicate her effort. Often, I waited for about an hour after her scheduled shift had ended for her to finish with her paperwork. Many other doctors mentioned time pressures, feeling like they did not have enough time to work on a case or "to go deep," and feeling "always on the run."

Donatas, a hospital administrator and doctor, expressed his frustration with the International Organization for Standardization quality-management standards that have been implemented in the Lithuanian health-care system: "We teach doctors to be prepared for an audit, observe the strict laws, follow all the protocols, and I manage them according to general management practices that come from the car industry or other industries. But in medicine you cannot predict every case! All these rules are not necessarily better for the patient. And the world turns a blind eye! It is very sad. Everyone works according to the protocols and for money." Doctors and administrators emphasized the pressure they felt to meet efficiency metrics that require shorter hospital stays and shorter waiting times. Lina, a cardiologist, complained, "My work is 20 percent doctoring and 80 percent administration."

Lithuanian doctors have become more efficient at curing, but not necessarily at caring in the way that patients want. Digitization and the standardization of procedures have not necessarily translated into more attentive or caring institutions. Patients complained about the lack of attention from doctors who looked more at the computer screens than at the patients and type. They perceived this typing—similar to the absence of a smile, a touch, a hug, or willingness to listen to life stories—as provocations and asking for envelopes.

Medical practitioners felt they were on the frontlines, facing patients' frustrations with being discharged from the hospital before they felt fully recovered, long waiting times, surgery quotas imposed by the State Insurance Fund, and other structural constraints.[8] Several of them referred to the general stresses that both patients and doctors experience. According to doctors, patients are "tired from life": exhausted and angry from working long hours, sitting in traffic jams, paying high heating bills, receiving small salaries and pensions, and experiencing loneliness. All these pressures made medical encounters more sensitive. The doctors were tired, too, from juggling jobs, families, and bureaucracies.

Lina repeatedly complained to me that patients underestimated the effort involved in a single patient visit. In particular, she was irritated when patients repeatedly knocked on her door after being asked to wait: "Patients do not interrupt hairdressers, but they do interrupt the work of doctors." (Quite a few doctors made this comparison.) "You say to them that the test results will be back in three hours, and they get annoyed. I tell them, come tomorrow at 8 a.m., and they say, 'I have to go to work,' or 'It will take me an hour to come from the other side of Vilnius.' They don't think about how much time it takes, and the work it takes to produce a diagnosis and treatment plan. When they come to this room, they want my full attention—I can't interrupt them when the appointment time is up and go immediately to the next patient. It takes what it takes. I wonder how they imagine our work—what it consists of. You should ask."

Almost all doctors talked about impatience. While sitting with patients in the emergency room and outside the offices of cardiologists and family doctors, I noticed that some patients would come in and ask to be seen before their scheduled appointment time. They would complain about long waits (though these were often no more than thirty minutes), talking to the nurses and doctors in raised voices. Some would not even say hello. The atmosphere of waiting rooms was emotionally charged. Patients suspected doctors of taking coffee breaks or chatting on the phone with their friends or families. While waiting, older patients exchanged complaints about their tough lives, politics, long waiting times, expensive medications, various supplements they were taking, their health conditions, their children, and the annoyances of the hospital (parking was tight, and some hospitals had started charging parking fees). I saw patients and their family members scolding doctors, and young doctors reduced to tears by patients' insults, but I never saw doctors or nurses yelling or raising their voices. Perhaps they restrained themselves because I was there, or perhaps it was because I was at one of the best hospitals.

The two decades of transformations alleviated some of the doctoring constrains such as lack of medication and technologies, or access to global medical knowledge. The new political economy opened up opportunities for research and learning. At the same time changes in health care posed different challenges to medical practitioners. These changes brought new management standards with its treatment protocols, efficiency, and emphasis on doctor's accountability, but it also increased the amount of paperwork and limited doctors' autonomy.

When Doctors Give

While I was doing fieldwork at the hospital, every morning I went upstairs to the cardiology unit and sat down on the red fake leather chair next to the nurses' station, which was a hive for doctors, residents, nurses, and patients. Facing the desk was a framed apostolic blessing from Pope John Paul II to the hospital staff. Sometimes his image seemed to be looking at the offerings of flowers, chocolate boxes, coffee, and gift bags from patients. That morning the pope was looking at white roses in a vase received from a discharged patient.

The unit can accommodate thirty-four patients at a time. They include unemployed people, pensioners, farmers, members of parliament, and CEOs of large corporations with various cardiovascular conditions, such as cardiac arrhythmias and aortic aneurysms. One day, two male patients were admitted to have pacemakers implanted to regulate their heartbeat. The unit performs approximately 800 such procedures each year. Sigitas was a tall man, a former track-and-field athlete, in his early fifties, and Petras was short and gray-haired, in his mid-seventies. They shared a two-bed hospital room. Both men were married to staff members in the cardiology unit: Petras's wife, Julija, was a veteran cardiologist, and Sigitas's wife, Violeta, was a nurse who often worked with Julija.

For the past two weeks, Julija had been telling her colleagues that she thought it was time for Petras to get a pacemaker. He had obtained a referral from a cardiologist at his local polyclinic and was scheduled for the procedure without the usual month-long wait. In the hospital, Petras was formally under the supervision of another doctor, not his wife.

Violeta had urged Sigitas, who also suffered from arrhythmias, to see a doctor, and he had become Julija's patient. After running some tests, she recommended that he get a pacemaker. It was a good time to do it, she observed, because of the current shipment of pacemakers. The previous one had made surgeons curse at the poor quality of the wires. A day before the surgery, Violeta seemed worried. She was anxious because she wanted Jonas, considered one of the best cardiac surgeons in the country, to agree to operate on Sigitas. Julija had already asked Jonas to perform the surgery on Petras.

It is quite common for patients and their relatives to do everything in their power to engage top-ranked or well-known surgeons (professors, heads of units, doctors who appear in the media). These surgeons were bombarded with requests to do routine surgeries when there were more complex cases requiring their expertise. Julija had already promised to approach Jonas on Violeta's behalf, but Violeta was asking other doctors and nurses in the unit for advice. "Should I go and ask him myself?" Violeta asked Linas, another cardiologist, who replied, "No, don't go. Jonas will think that you are imposing. He doesn't like that. Let our unit head do it. She knows him. And he will think that you care too much about a particular patient."

At lunchtime, Violeta and Julija were sitting at the desk talking. I sat quietly on a chair next to the desk with my notebook open, listening. Their conversation turned to the topic of envelopes. Violeta asked Julija, "How much should I give—200 or 300 litai at the beginning?" "Three doesn't look nice," Julija replied. "Give 200 at the beginning and then 200 at the end. I just gave exactly like this. You know, recently someone in our family needed a neurosurgeon. We gave him 400 litai, and he was very happy. Also, my sisters' husband had to undergo lung surgery in oncology; they called me and asked how much to give. 'We are thinking about 1,000,' they told me. I said: 'Give 700 litai now and 300 litai later, if you like the service. But it's not much for this kind of surgery, you know.'"

Even though Violeta and Julija were medical professionals themselves, this conversation about envelopes followed almost exactly the same script as stories I heard from other patients and family members. It had all the same elements: the concern to get the best doctor, worrying about the right amount to put in an envelope, comparisons with other people's illness experiences, and the doctor's opinion.

Finally, after all this waiting and suspense, Jonas came into the unit. He said hello to Julija and Violeta, asked "where?," took Petras's file and went into the patients' room. Julija followed him. Violeta was waiting outside. After ten minutes the surgeon left without saying anything. Violeta and Julija resumed their conversation at the desk.

> VIOLETA: Did he give money? [referring to her husband]
>
> JULIJA: He gave.
>
> VIOLETA: And?
>
> JULIJA: And nothing. Jonas said, "Thank you," and put money into his pocket. You know, next time, buy some sort of leather folder, a calendar, or something beautiful and expensive, and say, "This is for you, so you remember us." Now you will have to go back to him many times. Otherwise, you know, you put money into your pocket and immediately forget who gave it to you and how much.
>
> VIOLETA: It seems to me that it is a very normal amount, good for everyone, right?
>
> JULIJA: Uh-huh.

Violeta appeared satisfied that the amount her husband had offered was enough to indicate respect for the surgeon but still affordable for Violeta's family, but Julija seemed slightly disapproving of the way the envelope had been offered.

She was representing the doctors' perspective to Violeta and explaining how to make a payment seem more like a gift.

After a brief silence, Julija said to Violeta in a very friendly tone: "Look, we arrange things in three days for other people, so won't we do it for ourselves?! Others are taking pigs from farms, we also use what we can." Her last remark was puzzling. Initially I thought that she was making an ironic reference to the situation under socialism, and I attributed it to her age. But then Violeta took her hands out of the large pockets of her white coat and asked, "Did you see yesterday on TV how this woman was caught with twenty kilograms of sausages at a meat-packing plant?"

"No," said Julija, abruptly fixing her reading glasses on her nose and placing a patient's file on the desk.

"She wrapped all these sausages around her body and then put her coat on. But one sausage was hanging loose below the coat, so the security guard saw it. The guard stopped the woman to tell her that something was wrong, and he saw that it was a sausage," Violeta recounted.

"Poor woman," nodded Julija.

"Indeed, how unlucky," agreed Violeta.

I could not stop myself from interrupting the conversation at this point. I was not surprised that the nurse and the doctor were discussing envelopes, but I wondered how Julija's comparison between stealing pigs and giving envelopes had led to the topic of sausages. When she recounted the sausage story, Violeta did not use the words theft or stealing but rather taking away and appropriating. It immediately brought back my memories of life under socialism. It was common for goods such as food and clothing, car parts, and cosmetics to be appropriated from state-owned factories and sold by workers and managers. So, I was surprised to learn that these appropriations apparently remained part of daily life. After twenty years of capitalist development and private enterprise, modern security systems, and the implementation of new standards and work ethics, workers were still acting like it was the 1970s or 1980s. The flourishing of the informal economy and appropriations under socialism have been explained as the consequence of bad planning and constant shortages. How was it being explained now, when there was, if anything, an oversupply of sausages and other goods in the stores and supermarkets in Lithuania?

"Is that still happening?" I asked Julija and Violeta.

"What should the poor woman do?" Julija asked. She looked at me, adjusted her glasses again, and continued, "People are not paid properly. What can people do if they don't get paid? They have families to feed. People are oppressed (*spaudžiami*) like under the Soviets, maybe even more." She interpreted the episode as a challenge to capitalist exploitation and comparable to resistance to the socialist state.

To understand the current context of such activities, I asked them, "Do you get your salaries on time?" Violeta and Julia responded almost in unison, "Yes, we do." But, Violeta added, "We will have to take two weeks of unpaid leave. Our salaries will be slashed by 10 percent this year, and we only have funding until July 1." Julija continued, "And then we don't know, maybe we will have to work for free. The only people being treated here will be those returning from Ireland or England and paying us 100 litai."

"You, too, will have to pay to sit here," added Violeta.

Assertions of Good Doctoring

Enveloped care is situated in a context of temporal and material scarcity. Patients and doctors alike expressed a desire for more care—attentive and competent doctors, and respectful, cooperative, and compassionate patients—but doubted that this was possible given the constraints doctors work under. They assured me that even before applying to medical school, they knew that the worst possible conduct would be to anticipate payments and differentiate between patients based on how much they gave. At the same time, they expressed frustration over low pay and the restrictions placed on their professional judgment by time pressures and restrictive protocols.

This ethical regime allows space for the practice of enveloped medicine to shape particular forms of care. Doctors used the phrase "I am a doctor" to assert that monetary considerations did not affect their treatment decisions or their relationships with patients. Without exception, they swore that the amount patients offered did not matter to them, although they alluded to other doctors for whom it might. I take these assertions—"I am a doctor," "I am not asking," and "I do not want to sell health care"—not as statements of fact but as beliefs and assertions of a particular position in doctor-patient relationship. I draw on Michel de Certeau's concept of belief "not as the object of believing (a dogma, a program) but as the subject's investment in a proposition, the *act* of saying it and considering it as true—in other words, as the 'modality' of the assertion and not the content" (1984, 178). Thus, these statements are investments in enactments of what constitutes a good doctor. But they are also situated in a particular reality: doctors cultivate the appearance of being indifferent to money and yet are simultaneously dependent on it. They are caught in ambivalence. This, in turn, shapes the reality of health and care in Lithuania.

Julija and Violeta behaved similarly to many other relatives, yet they had the significant advantage of being medical practitioners. While in my presence, both women justified their actions as necessary for taking care of loved ones in unfair conditions, equating the state's neglect during socialism with capitalist exploitation today. They are exemplars of the will to care and caring collectives explored in the next chapter.

COLLECTIVE CARE
Relations of Obligation

"Here is my smoker," Jurgis smiled, pointing to a rusty box buried in the ground between the apple and pear trees in his backyard. He had lived in this small yellow house, on a quiet street in a regional town, since 1948. "I haven't used it for the last ten years. I could smoke again, I think, since I got this Mercedes [referring to his pacemaker] in my heart a year ago. I wanted to, but my daughter says that these days doctors can buy everything. There are plenty of things. It is better to give money."

Jurgis's daughter, Alma, was taking care of him, making medical appointments, and giving gifts to the doctors. "She knows how to do that," noted Jurgis, smiling and touching his heart. "Alma arranged the best doctor for me, the gifts, everything." Listening to her father, Alma smiled and nodded in agreement. "I do, Dad, I do," she said while picking fallen apples from the lawn.

Jurgis got the meat smoker in 1975, when his wife, Elena, was diagnosed with leukemia. He knew how to smoke ham and sausages, but he had wanted to start making smoked chicken, which was something out of the ordinary then. "During that time the stores were almost empty, selling chicken only from industrial collective farms, a bluish-violet color, skinny and tasteless, while my smoked chicken was the best. I was good at it," he told me. He also smoked eel, ham, and sausages, which he gave to the doctors and nurses to get friendly care. Alma was seven years old when her mother was diagnosed with leukemia. She remembered that Jurgis spent the next two years "nonstop smoking food, making food, and taking it to the hospital in Vilnius for both my mother and the doctors. My father loved and cared for my mother every way he could."

Jurgis started using food to care for his family long before his wife was diagnosed with cancer. In 1944, Jurgis was a young man in love. All he wanted was to marry and work on his ailing father's farm. If it had not been for the war and occupation, this dream might not have been so difficult to realize. In 1944, the German army retreated from Lithuania, and the Russians returned. Men like Jurgis were being drafted into the Soviet army and sent to the front lines to fight the Nazis. He had no desire to fight for a country that seemed alien to him: "I really didn't want to take any sides—to join the Soviet army or resistance movement. I just wanted to live my life."

Jurgis came up with a plan; he took smoked ham from the family barn, put it in his backpack, and set out to walk the eighteen kilometers to the town of Ukmergė. There he intended to find a doctor, give him the ham, and ask for a diagnosis that would exempt him from the draft. Then he could work on the family farm and marry his beloved Elena. His father gave him a golden coin, in case the ham was not enough to persuade the doctor. This 10-ruble coin, issued by Tsar Nicholas II, was all the savings his father had, and he had inherited it from his father. Jurgis was hoping to find the doctor who had saved his little sister from dying from pneumonia in the 1930s. (He came from a family of fourteen children; only he and three of his sisters survived into adulthood.) Even though Jurgis's family was short on cash—they could only pay the doctor with 1 litas and a dozen eggs—the doctor came out to their farm in the middle of winter on a horse-drawn sled.

Things did not work out the way Jurgis and his father had intended. Jurgis was arrested on the way to the town on suspicion of belonging to the Forest Brothers (an anti-Soviet resistance movement) and was imprisoned in Vilnius for three months. Eventually he did marry Elena, and they settled in Ukmergė. The family farm was nationalized, and Jurgis became a collective farm worker. The postwar years were tough. The state deported neighbors to the labor camps in Siberia and seized crops from their farms. In the cities, the situation was even worse. Besides working on a collective farm, Jurgis and Elena were rearing pigs in their small backyard and traveling sixty kilometers every Saturday to sell the meat in Vilnius. With their earnings they would then buy wool that they could spin into yarn to sell. "That is how we made a living when we no longer had our land," Jurgis told me. People engaging in this sort of small-scale commerce were known as "speculators" (*spekuliantai*) and ridiculed in the press (Klumbyte 2011).

Evading the draft through a medical diagnosis had seemed like a plausible way for Jurgis to care for his family. They bet almost everything they had on the plan. The potential bargain with the doctor, facilitated by food and money, offered a way to overcome hardships and to care for others, survive, and love in uncertain times. Such arrangements were common under socialism and, as we have seen, they persist into the present through the will to care.

Present in patients, caregivers, doctors, and nurses, this will reconfigures the terms of care and how it is measured. The will to care is not expressed by the conscious and calculated choice of an autonomous subject; it is immanent and relational, inseparable from collective obligations. For instance, in the case of Adomas's family, described in chapter 2, giving an envelope in the late 1980s was an expression of hope for a miraculous cure in the case of his mother's untreatable illness, even though she was against enveloped practices. Lucija also placed her hope of healing in envelopes. Alternatively, for Brigita and her aunt, it was a way to deal with the effects of anesthesia. For Justinas it was an expression of both—his goodness and gratefulness to the cardiac surgeon. Justinas disdained those patients who did not care and did not feel indebted to doctors. He perceived them as uncaring. Rasa, who took care of her aging parents, conveyed that giving envelopes allowed her to feel like a caring daughter. She and her siblings did everything they could so her mother would feel cared for. Rasa also felt empowered to ask questions and foster bonds with doctors, and advise others on how to navigate through the maze of the current health-care system. Whether during soviet socialism or current configurations of postsocialist capitalism, patients and caregivers dwell in webs of obligations that drive this will to care. Hence, it also opens possibilities to think about how care, generosity, and relations make inroads into medical settings.

Jurgis explained his reasons for building relationships with doctors: "When you have children, a wife, sisters, in-laws, and you and your wife are not getting any younger, you always need good and friendly doctors. . . . If I caught more fish on a weekend than I needed, I gave some to the doctors. I gave them food—meat, apples, eel. I lent them my car if they needed to go to the city or visit their parents in another district." Jurgis also gave money. "When the situation was more serious . . . you know, apples are apples, but doctors needed other things too," he said, rubbing his thumb and fingers together to suggest money. From his perspective, Jurgis was attentive not only to the needs of his family but also to those of doctors, from quality food to cars, furniture, imported shoes, or jeans.

For Jurgis, relations of care are expressed materially. Food, money, love, and obligations are interrelated. Elizabeth Roberts (2012), in her work on reproductive technologies in Ecuador, traces how relations of care—expressed in terms of time, money, and bodily attention—are involved in medical treatment. She explains, "Dollar signs fill some of the space between these relations, as well as the relations between doctors and patients, and doctors and equipment. Money makes it possible" (Roberts 2012, 5). Things construct relations and care; they make care visible and create caring doctors. Material things help facilitate relations of care, but according to Jurgis, they are not enough. Not all doctors easily accepted things, so instead he had "to come up with something interesting"—not just a chicken or some money, but a story, "to show that you care." One of the doctors, a cardiologist whom Jurgis remembered as "the best doctor" he had ever met, told Jurgis when he brought him a smoked eel: "Gifts will not help you, I will always help you, drugs will help you."

But the doctor was not right, according to Jurgis. Gifts and envelopes "changed doctors' personalities," making them friendly and "better" doctors. As I described in the previous chapter, all the doctors I interacted with said that envelopes had no impact on their decisions because they are doctors who help patients with their biomedical knowledge and the tools available to them no matter what. Yet they also acknowledged that once they accepted envelopes, they felt obligated to listen "to long stories about patients' lives, their children, and animals," which often helped them forget how exhausted they were from seeing so many patients and the "ton of things" they had to do. They needed those moments to "stop and smile." In other words, envelopes humanized care and made it more affectionate. This affectionate care is as important for Jurgis as biomedicine. He does not separate them, showing how he measures medical care based on affective (bio)metrics—his own feeling of what good care is.

I have known Jurgis's daughter, Alma, a forty-nine-year-old project manager for a state agency, for many years and frequently asked her for advice on navigating the medical system. She was less convinced about the importance of giving food or envelopes. For her, the competence and personality of doctors matter more than their friendliness. "Sometimes you give and nothing happens, you don't feel the effect," says Alma. Nevertheless, giving envelopes is such an integral part of life that she does not question it much. She does it mainly to please her father: "My father told me, 'You have to give, you have to thank the doctors.' There is no question for him." In the beginning, she did not argue because it made her father feel better if she gave to the doctors. "Later I tried to convince him that whether you give something or not, it doesn't matter. But no! My father believes in doctors, and that this is the way to get the best. . . . Then I simply accepted it." Alma gives to doctors out of obligation and love for her father, as many other caregivers expressed as well.

"My father often talks about this Mercedes in his heart," Alma said as we were slicing apples to make apple butter, "he picked it up from surgeon Jonas, who installed it." After the surgery, when Jonas came to check up on her father, he sat on his bed for a few minutes, asked questions, explained what had been done to Jurgis's heart, and even joked with him. Alma's father did not know that she had not given anything to the doctor yet. "You know, it was so hard to hunt down cardiac surgeon Jonas," she explained. When her father was hospitalized, it was not clear who would operate on him until the day of the surgery. That day, the nurses told Alma that Jonas might do it if there were no unexpected emergencies. According to her, it was their luck to get Jonas. When Alma went to his office before the surgery, he had already left for the operating room. "So, I waited till after the surgery and again he didn't show up . . . I was losing my patience . . . but I needed to thank the doctor, just in case, you know." The next morning, Alma waited for Jonas at his office, but again he did not show up. She only "caught the surgeon by chance" at her father's bedside when he was checking in on Jurgis. She followed the surgeon when he left the hospital room and, in the corridor, put an envelope into the doctor's pocket saying, "Thank you, doctor." The surgeon "looked at me and nodded, acknowledging it without any words," Alma recalled. She told me that she doubted whether the surgeon would even remember her, her father, or the envelope. But, according to Alma, the surgeon deserved "every litas," meaning all the money in the envelope, and Alma fulfilled her duty "to the cult of giving," as she joked. Alma embodies the ambivalence of giving envelopes; like many other patients she does it despite herself and her skepticism, expressing the will to care that her father instilled in her.

While the apple butter was simmering, Alma called her childhood friend Daiva, a widow who lives a couple of blocks away and works as a janitor in the local school, to invite her for dinner. Alma also asked whether Daiva by chance had made cheese (*Gal kartais sūrį darei?*). Judging by the excitement in Alma's voice, I gathered that Daiva was going to bring some of the excellent farmer's cheese she was known for. Daiva came in shortly thereafter, apologizing that she had only brought a small piece. She explained that she had given the bigger piece to her family doctor the day before. "It is the only thing I can give," she explained to me. She had conflicted feelings about giving it to the doctor. "You can't buy cheese like this in the store. Everything now has tons of chemicals. The doctor is very happy to see me with the cheese. She always looks not only at me but at my bag, too. She stares at my bag. I feel like I have to bring something."

Jurgis had been napping on the small sofa in the kitchen while we were making the apple butter. By the time Daiva arrived, he was awake and included himself in the conversation: "If you gave to the doctors and they helped you, treated you, why complain? I don't get it. You should be happy to be alive."

"Who says I am complaining? I am just talking, Uncle Jurgis," Daiva responded and then pondered the value of her gift to the doctor. "Maybe in Vilnius the cheese wouldn't be enough, Alma, you know, but here I get by."

Alma laughed and replied, "Oh, this cheese would be a success in Vilnius! Ask Elona if you don't believe me." Elona is a doctor who works in Vilnius and has been a classmate of theirs. Both Alma and Daiva call her for advice, and Elona also makes phone calls on their behalf and suggests which doctors to see. "But she never tells us how much to give. 'No amount is too small,'" is her typical answer, said Alma.

Daiva added, "She always tells me, 'Daiva, you don't have to give,' so I bring cheese or a chocolate."

"Elona is our health care system," Alma concluded.

Money is tight for Daiva, as it is for many residents of the area. She earns 750 litai per month after taxes (the minimum salary in Lithuania) as a janitor and considers herself lucky to have a job at all. Unable to keep up with the high heating bills for the apartment she had been living in on the fourth floor of a concrete Soviet-era building, she moved back to her parents' crumbling house after they passed away. To supplement her income, she grows vegetables and keeps chickens. Daiva's brother-in-law has cows, and every week he brings her a couple of buckets of milk. She inherited 5 hectares (2 acres) of land, which was converted to nonagricultural use to qualify for an EU compensation scheme aimed at controlling agricultural overproduction. With this money (400 litai per hectare per year) she began repairing the house.

Daiva showed us a new blouse she had bought in a secondhand market for 2 litai. "That is what most of us in small towns can afford. There are no stores selling new clothes. Nobody would buy them here. There are no jobs and no money." Facing such conditions, young people are leaving for Vilnius or other countries in the EU. Daiva's only daughter, twenty-two-year-old Monika, studies in Britain and supports herself working as a part-time cashier at Tesco and cleaning hotels.

From our conversation, I learned that Alma not only takes care of her father but also makes appointments for Daiva and takes care of her, too. Daiva, in turn, checks on Jurgis twice a day when Alma is in Vilnius. Later that night, after Daiva left, Alma told me that she had given small envelopes to the doctors on Daiva's behalf when the latter had to go to Vilnius for tests and consultations. Their doctor friend Elona had told her colleagues about Daiva's economic circumstances so that they would not have unrealistic expectations. Daiva does not know this. Alma says she does not want Daiva to feel indebted because Alma feels indebted to Daiva for taking care of her father.

Jurgis, his daughter, and her friends care for each other collectively and share their caring obligations. Here Jurgis's desire to give, Alma's ambiguity and trust in competent doctors, and Daiva's participation combine to enact enveloped care, which is driven by the will to care. Their circle of care widens to Elona, who is a classmate and a doctor. Elona, like many other doctors, is drawn to enveloped care by her obligations to existing and previous relations. That circle also includes friends and other family members. Despite all the doubt, this collective effort gives everyone involved a feeling of comfort and belief that everything will be all right. This collective, and others like it, is also a demonstration of the will to care.

Caring Collectives

For Alma, giving envelopes to doctors is a sign of her own care for her father, which she believes motivates doctors and nurses to care more about him as well. Another means of demonstrating caring is to inquire frequently about the patient's health. At the cardiology unit where I was observing, calls came in every day from the clinic administration, bureaucrats of the ministry of health, relatives, classmates, friends, neighbors, and other doctors asking for someone to be admitted to the unit and inquiring about the condition of certain patients, the surgery lineup, referrals, medications, and many other things.

Hospital staff, from doctors to maintenance workers, also came in person to ask about patients in the unit. These visitors often provided intimate details of patients' lives (recently divorced, a widow, an alcoholic husband, children living abroad, lost job, loves dogs, works the land, nervous, noncompliant with medications). Visitors asking about older patients and those from outside Vilnius often emphasized that the patient was not used to being hospitalized and might feel lost (it was easy to get lost in the building, a nine-story labyrinth with multiple units, diagnostic facilities, and surgery rooms).

These descriptions were not necessarily positive. Rather, they provided details of the patient's life that the visitors thought would facilitate better medical care and show that the patient was cared for by others. These caregivers also offered to help the doctors or nurses by talking to the patient about his or her condition, buying supplies, contacting relatives, or using other necessary connections. Sometimes they also brought gift bags to the doctors and nurses. Usually, the treating doctor would listen, quickly summarize the case, inform the visitor that there were no adverse developments, and promise to take good care of the patient. The visitor would nod and explain that they were obligated to ask and show interest, and then would go and visit the patient to recount their talk to the doctor.

Doctors from other units also came with gift bags and envelopes to talk to the cardiologists on behalf of their own relatives, as we saw in the case of Julija, Violeta, and other doctors. These encounters often involved more persuasion from the giver and resistance from the recipient. I happened to observe one of these interactions through the open door of the doctors' offices. An endocrinologist was discussing with a cardiologist whether her father should have a pacemaker inserted or just continue taking Cordarone, a drug used to control cardiac arrhythmia. The endocrinologist was pressing the cardiologist to say whether she would insert the pacemaker if it were her own father. The cardiologist paused for a minute and said, "You said that he is compliant with taking medications. Then I say, once you put something into the heart, you cannot take it out." "Thank you, this is what I wanted to know," the endocrinologist replied. And then she handed over an envelope, saying, "Doctor, this is for you. It is symbolic (*Čia jums, simboliškai, daktare*)."

"Stop it," the cardiologist said, raising her usually calm and gentle voice, "I am taking care of your father!" Her tone suggested that she felt the endocrinologist doubted that she was a good doctor. "No, no, that's not what I mean. It is an expression of collegiality (*čia jums kolegiškai*)," the other doctor responded. The next day her father was discharged to begin adjusting to Cordarone.

These visits and inquiries were so common that it was hard to tell whether they had any effect. Undoubtedly, personal stories about the patients supplemented their medical history; they also individualized the patient as a person with a certain life story and character, connected to a larger network of relations and caring friends and relatives. By contrast, doctors and nurses were annoyed by overly frequent inquiries, especially from bureaucrats. The staff would comment that instead of coming to visit and spending time with the patient, these officials only made calls. Nurses compared notes on Lithuanian politicians, discussing which ones were diligent about visiting their relatives and respectful and polite toward the medical staff, and which ones only called and made demands, showing off their power while simultaneously voting on austerity measures in 2009 that cut public spending for health care. Only a few high-level politicians were identified as caring. One of them had convinced a hesitant doctor to accept a thank-you gift by saying, "Who, if not people like me, can afford to thank you properly?"

Fielding all these calls, inquiries, and visits, with or without envelopes, also put pressure on the staff. One morning, after handling several calls and relatives in the cardiac unit, Lina burst out, "Is this a doctor's work? All these calls, all these requests, and people? No! It's not. I should be immersed in curing patients. That's what a doctor is supposed to do, not manage referrals, lines, attend to moods or desires. But I do it. We need to end this humanism." Clearly it was hard to manage calls from a variety of people, relatives, and all these intermediaries with her obligation to "simply cure" patients. Attending to the sensibilities of patients' social lives was not, according to her, a professional task. What the doctor referred to as "humanism" is the intertwining of scientific facts and health-practice protocols with personal values and expectations. Other doctors also expressed a desire to devote their time to medical science. "I don't have to do this," Lina said; yet she continued to do so. Doctoring in Lithuania is not limited to clinical work. Doctors are rewarded and recognized by patients and their family members not only for their clinical competence but precisely for exceeding these professional roles (Bazylevych 2010b). Obligations of curing and caring cannot be easily separated.

Doctors and patients are connected to larger collectives. As this book illustrates, the clinic is a nexus of a whole network of people, along with their pets and livestock, high heating bills, confusing hospital buildings, life stories, gift bags, envelopes, and health-care providers. Patients bring the whole bundle of relations to the clinic. Personalized ways of caring connect people to larger collectives of people and things (Puig de la Bellacasa 2010). The enveloped relation is multi-faceted, connecting not only a doctor and patient but also their family members, friends, and colleagues. Even though envelopes may appear to be an exclusionary practice, they are inclusive in the sense that they help to individualize patients, adding stories and personalities to the diagnoses, biomedical descriptions, and symptoms.

Patients' families contributed both practical and emotional support in the unit, constituting what Michael Taussig (1980, 8) calls the therapeutic milieu—the friendships and connections that patients develop during hospitalization that are important to the healing process. Sharing their experiences in a highly rationalized environment and helping each other allows patients to retain their personal autonomy while assisting and at times contradicting medical staff. However, the caring relationships I observed at Vilnius Hospital are much broader than the therapeutic relationships that Taussig theorizes. They extend to what I call caring collectives—relatives, neighbors, colleagues, medical practitioners—both inside and outside of the hospital setting. They are not necessarily intended to preserve a patient's autonomy but rather to emphasize the importance of interdependency. Nurses, for example, valued the help they received from relatives at the clinic: walking patients to the bathroom, feeding them, informing nurses that an IV needed to be changed, or clarifying the needs of older patients. Their presence was valuable when the unit was short-staffed. On weekdays in the cardiology unit, four or five nurses attended to thirty-four patients. At night and on weekends, there were just one or two nurses.

Some patients did not have anyone to call or act on their behalf. These patients received more attention from the staff if they were easygoing, had a sense of humor, or were good storytellers. For instance, one day Lina informed the nurses and residents in the cardiac unit: "I am admitting a new patient. Born in 1920. He saw Germans. He knows how to tell stories. I can sit next to him, listen and listen. His hair is white, and he has a white beard. He is real. Nobody will visit him, so love him." The white-bearded old man with messy hair was rolled into the unit in a wheelchair. His sweatpants were marked with yellow urine stains, and the smell of his unwashed body filled the air quickly. From his accent I realized that he was not from Vilnius. It was obvious that the patient lacked care at home and had to be washed and cared for in the unit.

Although most patients were eager to leave the hospital—and the medical staff, dealing with a constant shortage of beds, was happy to discharge them as soon as it was appropriate—some lonely patients, usually elderly, did not want to leave. Residents and doctors advocated for them, arguing that they should be allowed to stay because they were lonely or because they created a good atmosphere. No one advocated for rude patients or those unable to establish good relations with their fellow patients or medical practitioners. Nurses described relations with these patients as respectful but cold (*pagarbūs bet šalti*). When patients were discharged, nurses would simply bid those patients goodbye, whereas with the favored patients—whether because of their demeanor or their generosity, expressed with envelopes—they exchanged kisses and hugs and said things like, "Please come back."

In a sense, the hospital can be considered an extension of the family, or a caring collective. Patients often expressed a desire to be treated like a family member by forging a loving, caring, and committed relationship with competent doctors. Enveloped care is parochial, an attempt to establish notions of family and friendship in the field of health care. But doctors told me they felt conflicted about these expectations. One doctor, Donatas, expressed the dilemma this way: "Are we curing (*gydome*) patients or providing service? Is the person walking through this door a patient or a client? People want their doctor to be like a father, mother, or priest, to give his soul, and be present the whole day. But if a patient does not like something, he or she immediately becomes a client. This is confusing for both sides." Indeed, patients used the practice of giving to press doctors and cultivating friendly personal relationships. Patients also use envelopes to make doctors more attentive to their demands, at times testing the limits of doctors' authority.

One morning, when I was sitting at my usual spot at the nursing station and scribbling my notes, I overheard Violeta ask another nurse and a resident at the nursing station, "Did you see that?" She was referring to a large woman in high heels, with peroxide blond hair, bright make-up, and an oversized black bag who had just marched into a four-bed room of male patients. They nodded. "What do we do now?" Violeta asked, as her colleagues rolled their eyes. In a moment the same woman emerged from the patients' room proudly bearing a large chocolate cake with a red rose on top. The woman entered the nurses' office and handed the cake to them.

I recognized the woman, Galina, and guessed what would happen next. She was married to a patient of Regina's, a man in his fifties who was on the waiting list for a heart transplant and whom I had seen hospitalized twice in two months. He was a former alcoholic whose liver condition complicated his medical situation. Now he was heading to a rehabilitation facility near Vilnius, to which many difficult patients were transferred, for a two-week stay. On his previous discharges from the unit, his wife had brought in three homemade cakes—for the doctor, nurses, and nursing assistants—as a gesture of thanks. After the first time, Violeta had thanked her but said that it was "really unnecessary." Violeta explained to me that she thought the cake might take a toll on the family's budget—Galina did not earn much, the warehouse where she worked was cutting workers' hours, and her husband's disability allowance was very modest, while their heating bills were increasing.

When Galina had rolled her husband's wheelchair into the elevator, and the sound of her high heels had faded away, Regina, Violeta, and Jolanta, a nursing assistant, discussed the situation. "I don't know what to do with her. They will be back soon. I told her not to bring the cakes, even though they were so tasty. You know their situation. I feel so sorry for the wife," said Regina.

"I told her, 'Your life is hard, don't do that,' but she just doesn't listen," affirmed the nurse.

"She is a good baker. I gave her extra diapers," the nurse assistant added.

"I packed them an extra supply of medication, the one we get from a charity. Poor woman, she has to suffer because of that alcoholic," concluded Regina.

Baking cakes, gifting boxes of chocolate, filling envelopes with money can be seen as expressions of sincere gratitude and a way to cultivate relationships that exceed professional relations between health-care providers and patients. Though we could read this encounter as Galina trading cake for a bag of diapers, free medications, and compassion, the exchange is not what matters the most. Giving in this way might also be seen as an expression of care for the patient and their provider. In this case, it is clear that the doctors and nurses thought not only about the patient—Galina's husband—but about her well-being and personal situation too. The cake was indeed tasty, not too sweet, and not too rich. But even more memorable was how Galina and her husband's story was baked into it.

Gifts in the form of food or other objects are considered socially significant "signs of attention," while money in an envelope is often seen as a signal of bribery and depersonalized relationships (Ledeneva 1998; Patico 2004; Yang 1994). Alan Smart argues that money alone does not make an exchange a bribe; however, he asserts that bribes, disguised as gifts, belong to the realm of market exchanges and payments (Smart 1993, 400). Mayfair Yang (1994), who studied *guanxi* (personal connections) in China, points out that bribes do not build relationships; rather, the relationships between the parties precede the gift. In other words, bribes are not embedded in social relationships. Hence, the timing of an offering—before or after a relationship is established or a service is rendered—serves to define the transaction.

In some illness encounters in Lithuania, this temporal distinction does not apply; chronic patients like Galina's husband, Jurgis's or Rasa's parents are likely to make repeated visits to the hospital. Building on Alena Ledeneva's (1998) work on informal practices in Russia (1998), Michelle Rivkin-Fish's (2005) ethnography of maternal care in Russia contrasts "regimes of equivalence"—calculated actions, including payments and bribes—with "regimes of affection" based on bonds of friendship and mutual obligation, connections, favors, and gifts. Caroline Humphrey, in contrast to Ledeneva, takes a different approach and criticizes the exchangist notion of an "economy of favors" as missing vital characteristics belonging to favors. She argues that in monetized and "incompletely marketized" situations (for instance, education and medicine), favors can be both a transaction and a favor (Humphrey 2012, 33). She states that people's actions cannot be reduced to the logic of exchanges or investments in social or cultural capital; instead, "this is a moral aesthetics of action that endows the actors with standing and a sense of self-worth" (Humphrey 2012, 23). The exchange provides recognition as in the cases of Lucija, Rasa, and Galina. What it adds to the relationship is incalculable. Mauss (2000) has taught us about the ambiguous essence of the gift, with its congruence of calculative self-interest and disinterest. Anna Tsing notes that "not only do self-described gifts and commodities nestle beside each other, but they also incorporate each other's characteristics, change into each other, or confuse different participants about their gift-versus-commodity identities" (2013, 22). Market exchanges are also saturated with affect, social expectations, and obligations (Ferguson 2015). Envelopes, cakes, and smoked chicken cannot be neatly classified as gifts, or bribes, or commodities. They contain elements of all of these things, and they exceed them.

In my fieldwork, many patients and caregivers did not necessarily define doctors as their friends or acquaintances, but they did develop a kind of kinship, as in Galina's case. Lithuania is a country of less than three million people, where most of its inhabitants can be quickly linked to a good doctor who operated on their neighbor, relative, or classmate. This does not mean that doctors and patients are directly connected as friends, but that distant connections can be easily activated into caring collectives. What is important here is not the cultivation of the friendship per se, nor having the doctor as a personal friend but being in a friendly relationship. Some patients, like Daiva, did not even know that envelopes were given on their behalf, while others asked their family members "to settle accounts." Caring collectives are not necessarily stable compositions. They are assemblages that are activated, deactivated, and re-activated depending on the situation when different individuals are enlisted to care for the sick in the best possible way.

Time to Care

"I hate being dependent on these envelopes. I love being a doctor," acknowledged Tomas, a thirty-seven-year-old family doctor who works two jobs, at the university clinic and at a polyclinic in Vilnius. The newly built condominium complex where Tomas lives with his wife and young son stands next to gray and decaying Soviet-style apartment buildings of the kind that house many of his patients and colleagues. Most doctors in Lithuania are not wealthy. Many of those I spoke with lived in the same type of apartment buildings as their patients.

Tomas said he frequently thought about leaving Lithuania to work in Britain: "I asked myself, why I am working as a family doctor? I had good grades. Maybe I need to pass the exams to become an anesthesiologist and go abroad." Some of his classmates from medical school did pursue careers abroad, while others switched from doctoring to being pharmaceutical-company representatives. Tomas acknowledged, however, that he loved being a doctor and spoke warmly of his patients. He also felt he was keeping a promise he had made to his mother, now deceased, to become a doctor. Envelopes from patients made a significant difference to Tomas, supplementing his monthly salary by 50 to 100 percent. They also allowed him to help his father, who is retired, with his winter heating bills. "It is not the nicest way to get paid," he sighed, echoing other doctors I spoke with.

Tomas was convinced that the privatization of health care would improve his situation, making doctoring more honorable and less dependent on alms. When I asked him how that would affect his patients, Tomas paused and said he did not know. "But it's not even the salary that bothers me, though it is very important. It is time. I have only fifteen minutes for each patient," said Tomas. He has many older patients—pensioners with chronic conditions like high blood pressure and cardiovascular disease—who regularly come to renew their prescriptions, carrying their state-issued prescription books. "I get jars of honey and envelopes with 20–100 litai inside, and I am grateful for that. Don't get me wrong. I feel appreciated and needed," he said. But he felt a constant demand from his patients for more attention. "What my patients want is to talk. They want to tell me about their lives, cry, while I have other patients waiting in line and angry if someone stays longer, which they forget when they come in and want to talk. I wish I could spend much more time with them, but I have to fill out a ton of documents, and I can't multiply myself."

Many of Tomas's older patients were lonely. Their children are busy with their careers or live abroad and only send them money. Sometimes they hand him an envelope while saying, "It's from my son, who lives in London." Other times, Tomas said, "When emigrants are visiting their parents, they accompany them and stay, to talk to me. They hand me an envelope and say, 'Doctor, please fix my father, give him the best medication, so I can leave him alone until I come back.' . . . But what they need, these older patients, is companionship and attention. I love my patients, but I cannot be a son for them. I cannot solve their emotional lives, I only can medicate. The polyclinic shouldn't be a social club—it's a medical institution."

In the summer of 2012, I came back to Vilnius and met with Tomas in a café in the old town for a beer late on a Friday night. He looked tired and concerned. His father had suffered a stroke and was still in the intensive care unit at the university clinic. Tomas was confident that his father would recover, but now he faced another worry: "I am in the situation you are writing about. How can I thank the doctors?" When his father regained consciousness, he immediately asked whether Tomas had settled things with the doctors. Tomas told him not to worry. Now, sitting with me at the café, he pondered out loud: "It's difficult for doctors. You know, once one of my professors told us that we would get bribes, envelopes, and we should just get used to them, or difficulties would arise with other doctors and relatives. I was trying to approach the doctor, but he was running away from me, he was avoiding the situation."

"What about your sister?" I asked.

"She doesn't believe that this will affect us in any way, and she is right. I watched how the doctors and nurses work in the cardiology unit. They are extremely professional and caring. Do you believe that it could be different?" He asked me. I did not have the answer.

The notion of good care is not given or universal. In this book I have explored the complexities of enveloped care and showed how it has persisted through different social and political systems. Cultivating relationships between doctors and patients mediated by money, food, or other objects helped to sustain lives through tumultuous times of war, occupation, and radical political and economic changes. Enveloped practices are ambiguous, but they condition medical encounters and have effects on patients' bodies, relationships with medical practitioners, and the health care system. They have created a particular economy of health that still persists.

The process of making envelopes transparent by turning them into copayments and introducing new insurance regimes is part of the marketization of health care. Envelopes and copayments belong to different legal and ethical regimes, yet neither is inherently transparent. Both contain money, but they are not the same, even though both are meant to compensate for the provision of health care and to maintain life. The distinction between envelopes and copayments speaks to the notion of health and its ethical provisions. Replacing envelopes with copayments would reform the Lithuanian health care system, but it is doubtful whether this transparent but profit-oriented system would be more beneficial for the patients than the existing one that Lithuanians are so ambivalent about.

This does not mean that maintaining these enveloped practices forever is a solution either. They are historically constituted, so they will evolve or dwindle depending on the context. The main challenge is how to modify the existing health care system so that it becomes less of an assembly line and more attentive to the needs of the population. Such a system would retain a personal touch and some space for gratitude to exist without being swallowed by the market. However, for that to happen doctors need to be more conscientious and have more time for patients. Having enough time and sustaining individualized and empathic approaches have become luxuries that work against the prevailing logic of efficiency and rationalization in contemporary institutionalized medicine. The amount of paperwork that doctors have to do has further increased since the 1990s. Doctors in Lithuania hoped that computerized systems would free them from paperwork, but that did not happen, and not only because Lithuanian IT systems are poorly designed. Anthropologists showed how in the United States the implementation of electronic health records that aim to maximize the time doctors spend with patients are turning doctors into bureaucrats and transforming patients into digital entities "with standardized conditions, treatments, and goals without personal narrative" (Hunt, Bell, Baker, and Howard 2017, 403). Enveloped practices indicate a yearning for that personal narrative and caring connection that only seem to be more at risk as health-care systems get more technocratic and neoliberal. Enveloped care is an attempt to hold on to affordable, sensible, and personalized medical care.

Bittersweet

Albina, or Albinute, as the medical staff affectionately called her, came to the mental health clinic in Vilnius every day wearing the same skirt and one of her two cardigans, with a black scarf with red roses draped around her wrinkled neck. Each time she came in, often interrupting another patient's appointment, she took a few candies from the pocket of her blue or dark green cardigan and gave one candy to each of us: the doctor, a resident, and me, as I sat observing the consultation. One day a new resident, on her first day of work, asked Albinute, "Why are you giving these to us? You should eat the candy yourself, or give it to other patients."

"No!" she said loudly, "My sister gave them to me and said to give them to the doctors. 'Be nice and give them to the doctors,' that's what she always tells me.

Take it, my little doctor (*daktaryte*), take it and eat it." The resident took the candy and seemed hesitant to unwrap it. To be honest, they were not all that appealing after having been carried around in Albinute's pockets or hands. The young doctor looked at her senior colleague across the consulting room. The older doctor nodded and started to unwrap her candy. The resident reluctantly followed suit.

Only after the doctors had eaten their candies and spoken to her would Albinute leave. I also saw her giving candies to patients she liked. Her almost mechanistic, repetitive, and ritual way of giving candy, followed by conversation, mirrored implicit societal norms. The candy functioned the same way as envelopes, boxes of chocolates, cakes, brandy, smoked eel, paintings, or books. They fostered conversation and attentiveness, exposing the vulnerabilities of both patients and doctors and extending medical encounters. For the doctors, accepting this candy seemed to epitomize what it meant to practice medicine in the Lithuanian health-care system. It obligated them to touch, smile, hug, listen to stories, and be nice. The relations of care between patients and doctors are like that candy: bittersweet.

FROM LITAI TO EUROS

On January 1, 2015, the euro became the official currency of Lithuania, marking the final step in becoming European.[1] In the Lithuanian imagination, the euro set the country firmly within Europe and farther away from Russia. The Baltic states joined the euro club just as belief in the currency started to wane and despite the warnings about the negative impact of the euro on countries like Lithuania. Nevertheless, the country proudly let litai, which had circulated since 1993, retire. At that time, litai had replaced a temporary currency, talonai, often called "vagnorkės" (after the last name of the prime minister Gediminas Vagnorius, who introduced them) or "little animals" (because there were pictures of animals like bears, deer, and bison on the banknotes). Talonai had been introduced in 1992 as transitional money when the country withdrew from the Soviet ruble system but was not ready yet to return to the litai, the money of independent Lithuania (1918–40). At that time, inflation was so high that a doctor could receive a box of chocolates full of talonai that was not worth that much. The introduction of litai ended a period of high inflation and began a period of relative stability. Litai circulated flawlessly, and Lithuanians trusted them. In the beginning, litai were pegged to the US dollar (with an exchange rate of 1:4) and then repegged to the euro (1:3.45), when Lithuania started the accession negotiations with the EU. Even during the 2008 financial crisis, the government chose internal devaluation instead of devaluating litai by changing the exchange rate to the euro. Monetary nationalism prevailed, saving peoples' trust in litai (Norkus 2017).

In the lead up to the currency transition, I was curious how the euro would affect envelopes. In the aftermath of the 2008 financial crisis, doctors told me that patients started giving less. Patients' generosity shrank simultaneously with their incomes. I was waiting for the moment to see whether the change in currency regimes, the actual use of new banknotes with lower denominations, would impact the calculation of money in the envelopes. I viewed this conversion to the euro as a test for my observation that money in an envelope was not the same as a payment. It did not function based on the logic of the market, and patients had their own logic of giving or refusing based on their own calculations and aesthetics of giving.

Litai had been pegged to the euro at the stable exchange rate since 2002 (3.45 litai to 1 euro), so the change in banknotes was only aesthetic—the euros had different iconography and smaller numbers. As expected, the technical introduction of the euro went smoothly. Lithuanians were familiar with euros, so the transition was almost a nonevent, and they figured that the new currency was going to be economically and politically beneficial. Switching to the euro solidified Lithuania's place in the community of European nations, made travel more convenient, and made business transactions even more efficient. However, whenever a country introduced the euro, prices spiked. It happened in Latvia, Estonia, and before that in Italy and other countries. Lithuania was no exception. A year after the transition, a cup of coffee that I used to buy at a café for 2 litai had a price tag of 2 euros. Visits to a private clinic went up from 60 litai to 60 euros. These changes illustrated how, as Guyer (2009) argues, all prices are fiction. Prices are compositional, resulting from additions and subtractions. However, the logic of composition is not necessarily clear. Traditional explanations of prices as a result of market self-regulation, regulation, demand, and supply were not convincing to the public.

Many Lithuanians blamed greedy business owners, who used the euro to jack up prices and profits. As prices went up, the government even considered opening state-owned grocery stores and pharmacies to control the costs of basic food items and drugs to protect vulnerable populations. These ideas were quickly deemed expressions of longing for the socialist past and were not followed through.[2]

In 2017, almost everyone I talked to was still translating euros to litai. A young couple with two small daughters shared their outrage: "The country will be too expensive to live in soon. We are no longer shocked by Norwegian prices. Norwegian!!!!" (In Lithuania, Norway is considered an expensive country.) Lithuanians, like this couple, flocked to Poland, which does not use the euro as its currency, to do their shopping—mainly for groceries and medications. Social media was full of posts comparing prices in Poland, Germany, Norway, and Lithuania, and most of the comments on the posts expressed outrage.[3]

Once the euro became the only official currency in the country, I talked to Ona, a sixty-nine-year-old pensioner who lives in Vilnius. Ona was worried that she would have to give more to her doctors. She explained: "I used to give 50 litai to my family doctor or cardiologist once or twice a year. Now it is what—14 plus something euros? Let's say 15. But even that doesn't look nice. How can you give: 10 and 5? It is not a 'round' amount (*apvali suma*) and doesn't look elegant. So, I don't know what I am going to do. Should I give 50 euros? That would be 172 litai. It is way too much. Maybe I will give just once. Maybe I will give 20 euros or give nothing. Even 20 euros—that would be 69 litai, which is almost 20 litai more! It is too much. I will give only if something serious happens to me." The euros evoked memories of litai and encounters mediated by litai. That constant recounting of prices and comparisons between now and then vividly shows how money is "a memory bank" (Hart 2001). Money in the envelope represents memories of illness and humiliation, previous medical encounters, and hope. The euro disrupted the whole calculation.

Ona was confused for a while, so she did not give anything on her visits to the doctors. She was more concerned about the aesthetics and performance of giving. The 50 litai in her envelope—an orange-brown banknote with Vilnius cathedral on one side and Jonas Basanavicius, a doctor and the patriarch of the modern Lithuanian nation, on the other—does not translate to 15 euro (14.49 to be exact). These 15 euros seemed to me like a logical round up of the conversion from 50 litai. Yet, for Ona, it did not look nice in the envelope. Seemingly mundane, the money in the envelope was not that at all. The aesthetics of money emerged in numerous conversations throughout my fieldwork, but the euro just emphasized it more clearly. Patients preferred to give one banknote instead of two: 100 litai was better than two 50 litai notes; 125 litai was not better than 100 litai. The aesthetic properties of money in an envelope were as important as its actual purchase value, confirming that money is both an economically valuable thing and a visually aesthetic object (Shell 1995, 9).

After a year of using the new currency, Ona was frustrated that she had to be extremely careful about how she spent her pension. She explained to me that a bunch of dill at the farmers' market went up from 1 litas to 1 euro. Refraining from buying dill, a necessary ingredient for a Lithuanian summer staple—cold beet soup—was not an option. Ona stopped giving envelopes to her doctors until she could be comfortable giving 10 or 20 euros again. Envelopes were always a gratuitous extra for Ona. Euros deprived her of that extra. Ona calculated her envelope based on both her income and the aesthetics of money, affirming that the "perception of currency value is an affective and aesthetic matter" (Lemon 1998, 23). The euro conversion showed that the numerical value of money as payment does not equal the aesthetic value of money as an offering. At times, the aesthetics of giving is more important than the economic value of banknotes. Money designated for the envelopes is a combination of both: an amount based on the patient's calculations (reflecting affordability and illness circumstances) that is aesthetically pleasing.

Loreta, the family doctor, told me that when euros were introduced, her patients stopped giving for a while. Other doctors also told me that after the appearance of the euro they received significantly fewer envelopes. Seemingly, like Ona, they were perplexed about the offerings and took their time to figure things out. When I talked to Loreta in 2018, she admitted receiving envelopes with 5, 10, and 20 euros. She also received more produce: fresh potatoes, tomatoes, and dill from her patients' gardens.

Produce, flowers, and other things were fluidly interchangeable with the money in envelopes. In 2009–10 my interlocutors recounted their logics of switching from flowers and chocolates to money as a way of better attending to the needs of doctors and for practical reasons (doctors were getting too many chocolates, flowers do not last long, nor do they help doctors feed their families). Money was just another method of giving. In the euro era, it went in the other direction, from money to produce.

Produce was also an option for the patients whose doctors refused to accept envelopes. When her doctor at Vilnius Hospital refused to accept an envelope with 50 euros from eighty-six-year-old Janina, a former milkmaid on a collective farm, she was confused. Janina insisted on giving something to the doctor, so she figured a way around the refusal. She gave her daughter the very same 50 euros and instructed her to buy the largest turkey from a farm that was close to the village where she lived. Janina's daughter brought this huge, fresh turkey to the hospital and gave it to the doctor, telling him that he could not refuse the turkey from their village. "The doctor had to accept," Janina told me proudly.

The switch to the euro coincided with campaigns against corruption in health care. After years of criticism from TIL for not taking the problem of corruption seriously, the Ministry of Health directed public health institutions to create corruption-prevention programs in every outpatient and in-patient clinic in Lithuania. Some clinics printed announcements explaining that giving envelopes to doctors was considered a bribe and that by giving envelopes they had committed a crime. Usually these announcements hung on the information board behind the glass. Other clinics limited their message to the information providing phone numbers and asking patients to call when they encountered corruption. I spent hours observing one of these information boards. No one stopped to look at it.

Maria, a doctor who allowed me to shadow her during my research, gave me a leaflet that patients were getting upon admission to the clinic. The flyer, blue with a yellow sunflower in the background, was titled "Corruption Prevention" and read, "Dear client, I am asking you to not engage in informal payments or compromise your dignity and that of the doctors. If you encounter any expressions of corruption, please call the confidential phone line or inform the clinic administrators. Director." Along the bottom was a sentence that read: "Your smile is the best thank you." While I was reading the leaflet, Maria offered me a cup of coffee and a piece of chocolate from a box a patient had given her that day. "Too bad you won't meet Doctor Rita today. She went home after a long overnight shift at the ER. A patient of hers brought around ten kilograms of fresh potatoes from her garden. Rita couldn't take all the potatoes, so she shared them with us,"

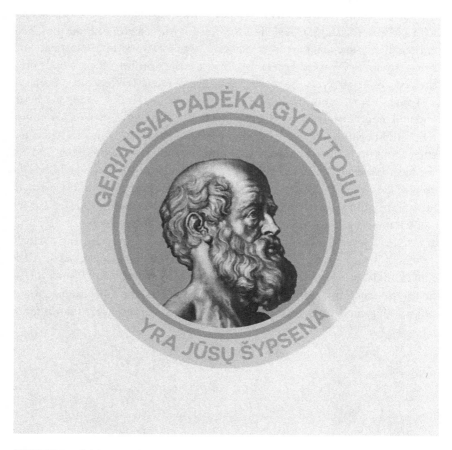

FIGURE 3   Sticker on the door of a doctor's office portrays Hippocrates. The surrounding text reads, "A smile is the best gift you can give to your doctor." Photo by author.

Maria explained as she pointed to a white plastic bag full of potatoes sitting in the corner.

Clinic directors were required to organize seminars for doctors and nurses to educate them on what a bribe is and what is acceptable. Many clinics had stickers with a similar message—that the best gift you can give a doctor is a smile or a simple thank you. These stickers indicate a shift from TIL campaigns that I described in chapter 1. The previous TIL campaigns relied on economic rationality. They tried to convince patients that "someone will always give more," hence the envelopes did not work. New campaigns recognize existing relationships between patients and doctors, modes of caring, and patients' desires to thank doctors. The stickers and leaflets aim to alter existing modes of giving: a smile instead of an envelope. Patients are encouraged to perform an emotion. Affect alone should replace material affective transactions.

In 2017, the doors at Vilnius Hospital and the outpatient clinic were plastered with stickers proclaiming, "A smile is the best gift you can give your doctor." I was curious about how well the new sticker campaign was working. "Do patients still bring envelopes?" I asked Loreta, who had a sticker on her office door. "Sure," she said, confirming that she continued to receive money, coffee, and chocolates.

I asked Loreta about the impact of the stickers. She smiled, shook her head, and told me a story about one of her patients, the grandfather of a former minister of health, who came in the day after every TV station in Lithuania had run a story about the anticorruption campaign and interviewed activists from TIL. "So the next day he comes in and gives me the box of chocolates. I say to him, 'Did you see the report on TV yesterday? I can't take anything from you.' He got mad: 'This is my gift to you from the bottom of my heart. None of those idiots on TV can tell me what to do, whether I can say thank you to my doctor or not! This is my gift. I never come empty-handed; I can't. You cannot refuse, my doctor.'" Another time, a patient tried to peel the sticker off the door. Loreta had to yell at him to put it back. He was angry: "They can smile on their TV, but I won't" (*Tegu jie ten televizijoje ir šypsosi*). Judging by Loreta's stories, the smile campaign was not working. Smiles are not something that Eastern Europeans are known for.

Notes

INTRODUCTION

1. Outside of medical settings, "little envelopes" are given as gifts for weddings, baptisms, and birthdays.

2. The reform projects also aim to fundamentally change the way health care is managed by instituting official copayments and introducing supplemental (voluntary) health-care insurance, while reducing the state's subsidies to the health-care sector. The documents use the words "nontransparent" income and "illegal copayments" synonymously, reflecting the tensions of shifting modes of rationalizing health care and articulations of the social in the postsocialist context (Healthcare Development Guidelines 2008–15 Lithuanian Ministry of Health [Tolesnės Sveikatos Sistemos Plėtros Metmenys, 2008–15]), Lietuvos Respublikos Sveikatos Apsaugos Ministerijos dokumentas, Lietuvos Respublikos Sveikatos Apsaugos Ministerijos dokumentas parengtas 2006 m. lapkričio 28 d. įsakymu Nr. V-1015 sudarytos darbo grupės. See also Healthcare Development Guidelines for 2011–2020 by Lithuanian Parliament (Lieutvos Respublikos Seimo Nutarimas dėl Lietuvos Sveikatos Sistemos 2011–2020 Metų Plėtros Metmenų Patvirtininmo, 2011 m. birželio 7 d. Nr.XI-1430,Vilnius), https://e-seimas.lrs.lt/rs/legalact/TAD/TAIS.401152/format/003_ODT.

3. Transparency International (TI) describes itself as "the global civil society organization leading the fight against corruption" and was founded in 1993 by the former World Bank manager Peter Eigen (Nuijten and Anders 2007). The Lithuanian branch of TI was established in 2000 under the auspices of the George Soros Open Society Fund of Lithuania.

4. I borrow the notion of healthscape as a "regime of practice" from Adele Clarke (2010).

5. "Will to care" is built on Joao Biehl's (2007) concept, the "will to live."

6. Ethnographies of health care in postsocialist contexts also described informal ways to obtain health care through both individual bodily practices as well as personal tactics to overcome existing conditions that nonetheless ignore structural injustice and undermine collective action (Brotherton 2012; Rivkin-Fish 2005). Yet informal payments are socially accepted, create new social relationships, and add affective value, functioning as an efficacy-affective form of redistribution and welfare functioning (Bazylevych 2010b; Morris and Polese 2014).

7. Created in 2006 by a group of residents led by the urologist Mindaugas Žiukas, this website, www.pincetas.lt, ranks doctors and health-care institutions in Lithuania, both public and private.

8. During my fieldwork the exchange rate between litas (LTL) and US dollar (USD) fluctuated between 2.4–2.8 LTL to 1.00 USD.

9. Here I draw from the friction between health as a universal notion (matters of life, biomedicine, standards, clinical trials, metrics) (Adams 2016; Cooper 2012; Dumit 2012; Kaufman 2015; Sunder-Rajan 2008) and care as particular (biographical, lived) (Biehl 2007; Das and Han 2016; Farquhar and Zhang 2012; Fassin 2009; Garcia 2010; Han 2012; Stevenson 2012) in contemporary anthropological studies of medicine.

10. In postsocialist Eastern Europe, the discourses of transparency, accountability, efficiency, and standardization overlap with the spread of neoliberal governmentality and are constructed vis-a-vis inaudibility, immorality, social networks, corruption, and the socialist past (Dunn 2005,168). After the Cold War, transparency has been lingua franca and has framed the ethics of neoliberalism (Ballestero 2012; Hetherington, 2011; Haller and Shore 2005; Sanders and West 2003; Strathern 2000a, 2000b). It has become one of the euphemisms of good governance, progress, and an open-market economy in the New World Order. Transparency is directly linked to the idea of the rational individual, yet "the individual is the true black box of transparency" (Hethertington 2011, 243). Often the absence of transparency is used to explain all failures (Morris 2004). Anthropologists showed that transparency does not necessarily make things less obscure and is also full of ambiguities (Ballestero, 2012).

11. Lucija was expressing the majority view. In multiple surveys conducted in Lithuania, 58.9 percent respondents opposed official copayments (Miškinis, Riklikiene, Kalėdienė, and Jarašiūnaitė 2011).

12. Health Care Development Outline 2008–15, draft of Ministry of Health of the Republic of Lithuania.

13. Lietuvos Korupcijos Žemėlapis, 2001–5, 2007, 2008, 2009, 2011, 2014, 2016 by Transparency International Lithuania. Corruption Maps for 2011–16 were commissioned by Lithuanian Special Investigation Unit, https://www.transparency.lt/lietuvos-korupcijos-zemelapis/.

14. L. Murauskiene, R. Janoniene, M. Veniute, E. van Ginneken, and M Karanikolos, "Lithuania: Health System Review," *Health Systems in Transition* 15, no. 2 (2013), https://www.euro.who.int/__data/assets/pdf_file/0016/192130/HiT-Lithuania.pdf, xviii.

15. All informants' names have been changed. I recorded some interviews, but mostly I took notes. Most of the interviews were conducted in Lithuanian. Some of my informants were Lithuanian Poles and Lithuanian Russians; I interviewed some of them in Russian.

16. The human economy refers to the economy made and remade by people. It is organized informally and dwells in the cracks of the economic system (Hart, Laville, and Cattani 2010, 1–17).

INTERLUDE I

1. Other stories circulate about doctors who receive bottles of brandy and cakes and sell them for cash. However, these stories do not have the same variety of versions and plots. Sometimes they are comments on the tales about boxes of chocolates. Perhaps the physical form of the box and the envelope, each capable of concealing other things, makes them more appealing as subjects, and objects, of storytelling.

1. FROM BRIBES TO COPAYMENTS

1. *Global Corruption Report 2006*; Transparency International 2006, 62. https://www.transparency.org/en/publications/global-corruption-report-2006-corruption-and-health.

2. Health Care Development Outline 2008–15, Ministry of Health of the Republic of Lithuania.

3. Korupcijos žemėlapis 2011, Vilnius. https://www.transparency.lt/wp-content/uploads/2015/10/korupcijos_zemelapis_20111.pdf

4. In 2009–10 approximately half of the patients engaged in informal payments in Lithuania (17 percent in primary care, 48 percent in hospitals). On average, patients spent 462 litai yearly; the medium monthly salary was 1,614 litai. Poor patients paid less than well-off ones or did not pay at all. The education of the patients was not a defining factor (Murauskiene 2013).

5. In 2016, the Association of Private Health Care Organizations conducted a study inquiring why patients were thanking doctors. The study did not use the language of bribery. According to the study, 51 percent of the patients hoped to get better care, 48.2 percent felt a moral obligation to give, 8 percent wanted to thank them because doctors' salaries were low, 11 percent decided to thank the doctors because they saw the patient sooner, and 13.4 percent felt "provoked." BNS, "Iš davusių medikui kyšį dauguma sako jautėsi moraliai įsipariegoję," http://www.delfi.lt/news/daily/lithuania/is-davusiu-medikui-kysi-dauguma-sako-jautesi-moraliai-isipareigoje-atsidekoti.d?id=73465336.

6. According to "the corruption map of 2014," 55 percent of the population thought that health care institutions were the most corrupt of all sectors of government. It does not provide the reasons behind these responses. The map's "bribery index," compiled from the indexes of "extortion, giving and effectiveness," reveals that the level of bribery in emergency rooms and in the Catholic Church (the respondents were asked where they felt they were being asked to give money) are similar,'" with polyclinics are not far behind. The "bribery index" at the hospitals is three times higher than in churches, Lieutvos Korupcijos Žemėlapis, "Visuomenės nuomonės tyrimų centras 'Vilmorus,'" n.d., https://www.stt.lt/analitine-antikorupcine-zvalgyba/lietuvos-korupcijos-zemelapis/7437.

7. The president of the Lithuanian Doctors' Union underscored multiple times the difference between the gift and the bribe. According to him, if doctors do not ask or there is no previous agreement about money or things then when patients give, it is a gift and not a bribe. LRT Televizijos Laida, "Kyšiai medicinoje: vis dar problema ar tik sąvokų painiojimas?" August 5, 2017, https://www.diena.lt/naujienos/kriminalai/nusikaltimai/kysiai-medicinoje-vis-dar-problema-ar-tik-savoku-painiojimas-823413.

8. I chose to show the video to the teachers and staff members of the preschool because their salaries were lower than those of the medical practitioners, and they did not live in the capital.

9. The World Health Organization considers Lithuania to have a moderate level of unmet needs and little difference between income groups; affordability is a challenge because of the high out-of-pocket cost for pharmaceutical drugs. At 2.9 percent, unmet medical needs due to cost, waitlist, or travel distance are below the EU average. In the poorest quartile, unmet medical needs due to cost are 1 percent in Lithuania versus 4.1 percent in the EU because of the lack of user fees for basic services and broad coverage. There were relatively small differences between income groups in reported unmet needs. "State of Health in the EU: Lithuania, Country Health Profile 2017," https://www.euro.who.int/__data/assets/pdf_file/0010/355987/Health-Profile-Lithuania-Eng.pdf, 12–13.

10. K. Prunskienė, "Išeitis Lietuvos ateičiai—socialinės rinkos eknomomika," Politikų Tribūna, TV3, November 17, 2009, https://www.tv3.lt/naujiena/lietuva/k-prunskiene-iseitis-lietuvos-ateiciai-socialine-rinkos-ekonomika-n319627.

11. Biopolitics here is understood as the politics of life, which emphasizes that populations are constituted as they are managed. For Foucault (2008, 317) biopolitics and market are intrinsic.

12. Z. Voitulevičiūtė, "Ar gydytojams tikrai pakanka dėkingumo šypsenu?" VL Medicina, April 29, 2012, http://www.vlmedicina.lt/spausdinimas//lt/ar-gydytojams-tikrai-pakanka-dekingumo-sypsenu.

13. Liutauras Gudžinskas, "Lietuvos ir Estijos Sveikatos Apsaugos Raida: Panašios Sąlygos, Skirtingi Rezultatai," Politologija 3, no. 67 (2012): 64. The divergence in health indicators started in the 1960s, when life expectancy in the Soviet Union began to stagnate (Roberts, Karanikolos, and Rechel 2014, 9). By 2012, many post-Soviet countries doubled the percentage of their GDP spent on health care, yet life expectancies in the countries of the former Soviet Union still lag far behind those in Western Europe. Lithuania's health-care spending (as a share of GDP) increased from 5.4 percent in 1995 to 6.6 percent in

2011 (Murauskiene, Janaoniene, Veniute, van Ginneken, and Karanikolos 2013, 43). Life expectancy in Lithuania, as in the other Baltic States, is lower than in core EU countries, but it is higher than in other post-Soviet countries. In Lithuania, life expectancy kept steadily increasing from 57.2 years in 1950 to 71.26 in 1969, and then held steady for almost the decade before going down slightly. It decreased from 70.83 in 1989 to 69.84 in 1994, and then kept steadily increasing to 71.86 in 2008 and 75.95 in 2020 (*State of Health in the EU. Lithuania: Country Health Profile* [Paris: OECD, 2017], https://www.euro.who.int/__data/assets/pdf_file/0010/355987/Health-Profile-Lithuania-Eng.pdf).

14. Lithuania's reform was based on Germany's Bismarck model, involving a universal health insurance scheme funded by business taxes and payroll deductions and a combination of public and private health-care providers. The first version of the proposal, drafted in 1992, was sent to reviewers in Germany.

15. D. Likaitė, E. Čeponytė, and V. Nakrošis, *Asmens Sveikatos Proežiūros įstaigų tinklo restrktūrizavimas 2008–2012 metais: Kaip pavyko trečias etapas? Kada reformos virsta pokyčiais? Politinis dėmesys, palaikymo koalicijos ir lyderystė A.Kubiliaus vyriausybės veiklos 2008–2012 metų laikotarpiu* (Vilnius: Vilniaus Universiteto Leidykla, 2015).

16. Lithuania has more practicing doctors (366.2 per 100,000 population) than the average for EU states (321.62 per 100,000 population) or the United States (24 per 10,000 population). It also has more hospitals than the EU average (3.36 per 100,000 population compared to the EU average of 2.97, and more than twice the ratio of Norway, Denmark, or the United States) ("Physicians per 100,000 People, by Country," Infoplease, n.d., https://www.infoplease.com/world/health-statistics/physicians-100000-people-country; "Physicians per 100,000," World Health Organization, n.d., https://gateway.euro.who.int/en/indicators/hfa_494-5250-physicians-per-100-000/). The number of practicing doctors remained fairly constant from 2005 to 2014 and even slightly increased in 2014, to 46.1 doctors per 10,000 people. The higher numbers are due in part to the 30-percent increase in medical residents (Oficialiosios statistikos portalas, "Medicinos darbuotojų dieną minint," April 27, 2015, https://osp.stat.gov.lt/informacin-iai-pranesimai?eventId=64821). By 2015, the number of hospital beds had decreased by 3.5 percent (Rita Gaidelytė, Milda Garbuvienė, ir Neringa Madeikyt, *Lietuvos gyventojų sveikata ir sveikatos priežiūros įstaigų veikla* [Vilnius: Higienos Instituto Sveikatos Informacijos Centras, 2015], https://www.hi.lt/lt/lietuvos-gyventoju-sveikata-ir-sveikatos-prieziuros-istaigu-veikla-2013-m.html).

17. Romualdas Buivydas, Gediminas Černiauskas, Liubovė Murauskienė, ir Robertas Petkevičius, *Lietuvos sveikatos priežiūros sistema pereinamuoju laikotarpiu: PHARE sveikatos priežiūros reformos projektas* (Vilnius: Sveikatos ekonomikos centras, 1997), 37, https://www.lsmuni.lt/cris/handle/20.500.12512/60655.

18. G. Budvytienė, "Širdies chirurgijos centras bus parduotas," *Kauno Diena*, June 2, 2003, https://www.delfi.lt/news/daily/lithuania/sirdies-chirurgijos-centras-bus-parduotas.d?id=2416969.

19. When Lithuania applied for EU membership, its health care had to be evaluated according to EU standards.

20. BNS, "Naujosios Vilnios gyventojai vėl kelia triukšmą dėl politklinikos," August 19, 2005, https://www.delfi.lt/sveikata/sveikatos-naujienos/naujosios-vilnios-gyventojai-vel-kelia-triuksma-del-poliklinikos.d?id=7313506; Lietuvos Profesinių Sajungų Konfederacija, "Nepatenkinti savivaldybės sprendimais dėl N. Vilnios ir Karoliniškių poliklinikų privatizavimo profsąjungininkai planuoja mitingą konstitucijos aikštėje," June 22, 2006, https://www.lpsk.lt/2006/06/22/nepatenkinti-savivaldybes-sprendimais-del-n-vilnios-ir-karoliniskiu-polikliniku-privatizavimo-profsajungininkai-planuoja-mitinga-konstituci-jos-aiksteje/.

21. "Mapping of the Use of European Structural and Investment Funds in the 2007–2013 and 2014–2020 Programming Periods," ESIF for Health, January 15, 2016.

22. Lietuvos Sveikatos Apsaugos Ministerija, "Antrojo Sveikatos Priežiūros restruktūrizavimo etapo ataskaita," 2009, https://sam.lrv.lt/uploads/sam/documents/files/Veiklos_sritys/II-ojo%20etapo%20ataskaita.pdf.

23. "Antrojo Sveikatos Priežiūros restruktūrizavimo etapo ataskaita," 3.

24. There were 15,229 beds in the state-run hospital, and 123 in private clinics. Lietuvos Respublikos Vyriausybė, "Nutarimas Dėl Ketvirtojo Sveikatos Sistemos Plėtros ir Ligoninių Tinklo Konsolidavimo Etapo Plano Patvirtinimo," Vilnius, December 9, 2015, https://www.e-tar.lt/portal/lt/legalActPrint?documentId=e6d81660a33a11e58fd1fc0b9bba68a7.

25. This is the basic amount used to calculate wages for state politicians, judges, civil servants, and public officers. The Ministry of Social Security and Labor defines main social indicators, including the basic amount, and updates them on its website. Lietuvos respublikos socialinės apsaugos ir darbo ministerija, "Pagrindiniai socialiniai rodikliai," January 26, 2022, https://socmin.lrv.lt/lt/veiklos-sritys/socialine-statistika/pagrindiniai-socialiniai-rodikliai.

26. BNS, "Medikams siūloma uždrausti iš pacientų imti net ir simbolines dovanas," April 4, 2005, https://www.delfi.lt/sveikata/sveikatos-naujienos/medikams-siuloma-uzdrausti-imti-net-simbolines-dovanas.d?id=6398982.

27. J. Paškauskas, "A. Čaplikas: Sveikatos apsaugai reikalingos reformos," *Bernardinai*, December 12, 2008, http://www.bernardinai.lt/index.php?url=articles%2F89171.

28. D. Jonušienė, M. Augustinaitytė, and A. Žukas, "Balto chalato kišenėse telpa daug," *Veidas*, December 3, 1998.

29. V. Kazakevičius, "Pacientai Lietuvoje jaučiasi diskriminuojami," *Veidas*, November 15, 2010, 47.

30. Sixty percent of Lithuanians were against any copayments for health care, according to a representative poll conducted in 2010 (R. Buivydas, G. Černiauskas, M. Schneider, and D. Zaleckienė, *Papildomo savanoriško sveikatos draudimo analizė* [Vilnius: UAB Sveikatos ekonomikos centras, 2010]). In 2013 only 17 percent of respondents were in favor of copayments, according to a poll commissioned by the Lithuanian Ministry of Health and conducted by "Baltijos Tyrimai." Elta, "Maždaug ketvirtadalis pacientų prisipažįsta davę kyšį," *Vakarų Ekspresas*, October 24, 2013, https://www.ve.lt/naujienos/sveikata/sveikata/mazdaug-ketvirtadalis-pacientu-prisipazista-dave-kysi/?utm_source=susije&utm_medium=referal&utm_campaign=blokas.

31. Lietuvos Korupcijos Žemėlapis, 2001–8, 2011–16, https://www.transparency.lt/lietuvos-korupcijos-zemelapis/.

2. BEING CAUGHT

1. Often the bewitcher is a neighbor.

2. In her article "On Key Symbols," Sherry Ortner examines the notion of "key symbol" as a mode of operation, thought, and action. Dominant symbols have elaborating power for conceptualizing the world and complex actions. Ortner argues that these key symbols "collapse complex experiences" that link individuals to the whole system (1973, 1340–44).

INTERLUDE III

1. Here I understand therapeutics as ethics, as defined by Cristiana Giordano (2014).

3. "I AM A DOCTOR"

1. The website Pincetas (tweezers) is a searchable database of doctors and health care institutions; it also allows patients to rank their doctors and for doctors to rank their colleagues. Doctors and patients have to fill out slightly different questionnaires. At the time of my fieldwork (2009–10), patients were asked to evaluate a doctor's professionalism,

communication skills, and caring attitude on a five-point scale. They were also asked about waiting times and payments—first about the official price of the consultation (ranging from free to more than 200 litai) and the value of gifts (*dovanos*) given to the doctor (from zero to more than 500 litai). There was a separate field for comments.

The questionnaire for doctors asks them to evaluate their colleagues' professional competence, theoretical knowledge, and ability to make clinical decisions; their ability to communicate with patients and colleagues; and their level of empathy and care for the patients. Lastly, doctors are asked to evaluate the actual price of their colleagues' consultations, and whether it is objective with regard to the patients' well-being. This questionnaire includes no questions about gifts.

The majority of the doctors that I observed in my fieldwork are listed on this website. Most comments rank surgeons as "good." Specialists (such as cardiologists) have more negative comments than surgeons. Most family doctors received equally good and bad comments. Unfavorable comments included "arrogant," "very strict," "uses ugly tricks," "unpleasant voice," "angry," "could smile more and not look so serious," and "doesn't come to see patients after surgery." Good comments included "being a doctor for her is a vocation," "a doctor that heals not only with the body but the soul, too," and so on. Some patients offered both positive and negative comments for the same doctor, such as "good doctor" and "money money money," or "first impression—pleasant" and "loves money." The percentage of patients who rewarded doctors with "gifts" varied from 20 to 50 litai, depending on the type of doctor. The typical amounts were up to 100 litai for family doctors and 100–300 litai for cardiologists, surgeons, and other specialists. Cardiac surgeons, according to the website, received up to 500 litai. In 2014, the website announced plans to remove information about the value of gifts because "averages don't have practical information for the patients" ("Mindaugas Žiukas: maždaug penktadalis pacientų prisipažįsta neoficialiai atsilyginę gydytojui," 15MIN, April 7, 2014, http://www.15min.lt/naujiena/aktualu/lietuva/mindaugas-ziukas-mazdaug-penktadalis-pacientu-prisipazista-neoficialiai-atsilygine-gydytojui-56-417922).

2. In 2009, paid sick leave was significantly limited. For shorter leaves (three to seven days), individuals were eligible for 40 percent of their earned income; for leaves of longer than seven days, they received 80 percent of their earned income.

3. Biological citizenship is necessarily connected to the political economy as recognition and hope for a better life for immigrant populations (Tickin 2006). According to Miriam Ticktin, "Biology is the domain of possibility and of hope, just as it is for those designated modern liberal subjects" (Ticktin 2006, 147). Biology as a means of manipulation is linked to modern sensibilities and the figure of the modern liberal subject, where biological citizenship is tied up with responsibility for one's biology (Rose and Novas 2005).

4. Biological citizenship became a basis for social membership, a new form of citizenship that emerged along with new structures of governance (Petryna 2002; Philips 2011), leading transitions of formerly socialist countries. In post-Chernobyl and post-Soviet Ukraine, the juridical status of the sufferer allowed one to access disability benefits during times of turbulent transition from socialism. In some cases, diagnoses that led to the status of disabled were the result of elaborate, illicit exchanges (Petryna 2002, 143). Events like Chernobyl can amplify the scope of tactics that had already existed.

5. Doctors' incomes are much lower than in the United States and Western Europe. Doctors are not associated with the rich in Lithuania, yet their salaries are like those of other professionals.

6. Regina was referring to a significant reduction in death rates. Between 1981 and 2010, the death rate from cardiovascular diseases dropped from 567 per 100,000 to 495

per 100,000; death from ischemic heart diseases decreased from 417 per 100,000 to 313 per 100,000.

7. These were largely well-known pharmaceutical companies such as Pfizer, Elly Lilly, AstraZeneka, and others. Doctors who worked in clinical trials expressed satisfaction with their pay and pride in participating in the research and working with the newest medications. Some of the doctors were opinion leaders in their fields and were paid for their talks to other doctors by these companies. Representatives of pharmaceutical companies visited quite regularly bringing lunches and talking about new drugs. The pharmaceutical companies also funded seminars and trips to international conferences. For more on clinical trials in Eastern Europe, see Pteryna (2009).

8. The number of surgeries depends on funding allocations from the State Insurance Fund (SIF). For instance, the number of state-funded hip replacement surgeries that can be performed depends on how many hip joint replacement parts that SIF buys and distributes each year.

EPILOGUE

1. The virtual form of the euro was born in 1999, and the actual currency began to circulate in 2002. In Europe, the euro symbolized the birth of a new social and political order (Hart 2005).

2. Jūratė Šovienė, "Valstybines vaistines: Kodel gi ne?" *Verslo Žiniso*, October 27, 2016, https://www.vz.lt/sektoriai/prekyba/2016/10/27/valstybines-vaistines-kodel-gi-ne; R. Valatka, "Lietuvoje regime kai kurių viduramžiško užsidegimo apraiškų," Dešimt minučių su Rimvydu Valatka," *Žinių Radijas*, October 31, 2016, https://www.ziniu radijas.lt/laidos/desimt-minuciu-su-rimvydu-valatka/r-valatka-lietuvoje-regime-kai-kuriu-viduramzisko-uzsidegimo-apraisku?video=1; R. Valatka, "Ko politikai nezadejo ir nezada," Dešimt minučių su Rimvydu Valatka, *Žinių Radijas*, February 25, 2019, https://www.ziniuradijas.lt/laidos/desimt-minuciu-su-rimvydu-valatka/ko-politikai-nezada-ir-niekada-nezadejo?video=1.

3. I. Janauskienė, "Pusmetis po euro: Brango viskas ar ne?" LRT, September 8, 2015 https://www.facebook.com/LRT.LT/posts/10154109462759129/; "Prices in Poland" (Kainos Lenkijoje) group, Facebook, https://www.facebook.com/groups/808296815981566/; Naglis Puteikis, post on the price of cauliflower, May 10, 2016, Facebook, https://www.face-book.com/puteikis?fref=search&__tn__=%2Cd%2CP-R&eid=ARBR4ZCSPEw5VJW-ZmXgC24ElS5VCT2Ob7EO0Xn7KscFJK9QiT3u796CqaTLnlZhWQdYwybgpr0jmLdvL; "Mikutavicius isklojo viska ka, ka galvoja apie lietuviskas kainas," Delfi, April 28, 2016, https://www.delfi.lt/veidai/zmones/m-mikutavicius-isklojo-viska-ka-galvoja-apie-lietu-viskas-kainas.d?id=71122552.

References

Adams, Vincanne. 1998. *Doctors for Democracy: Health Professionals in the Nepal Revolution.* Cambridge: Cambridge University Press.

———. 2016. "Metrics of the Global Sovereign: Numbers and Stories in Global Health." In *Metrics: What Counts in Global Health*, 1–19. Durham: Duke University Press, 1–19.

Aidukaite, Jolanta, Natalija Bogdanova, and Arvydas Guogis. 2012. *Gerovės valstybės kūrimas Lietuvoje: mitas ar realybė?* Vilnius: Lietuvos socialinių tyrimų centras ir Sociologijos institutas.

Andaya, Elise. 2009. "The Gift of Health. Socialist Medical Practice and Shifting Material and Moral Economies in Post-Soviet Cuba." *Medical Anthropology Quarterly* 23, no. 4: 357–74.

Ballestero, Andrea S. 2012. "Transparency in Triads." *PoLAR* 35, no. 2: 160–66.

Barthes, Roland. 1972. *Mythologies.* New York: Hill and Wang.

Bazylevych, Maryna. 2009. "Who Is Responsible for Our Health? Changing Concepts of State and the Individual in Post-Soviet Ukraine." *Anthropology of East Europe Review* 27, no. 1:65–75.

———. 2010a. "Negotiating New Roles, New Moralities: Ukrainian Women Physicians at a Post-socialist Crossroad." PhD diss., State University of New York at Albany.

———. 2010b. "Prestige Concept Reconsidered. Hybridity of Prestige in Post-Socialist Biomedical Profession." *International Journal of Social Inquiry* 3, no. 3: 75–99.

Bear, Laura, Karen Ho, and Anna Tsing. 2015. "Gens: A Feminist Manifesto for the Study of Capitalism." *Cultural Anthropology*, March 30. https://culanth.org/fieldsights/652-gens-a-feminist-manifesto-for-the-study-of-capitalism.

Biehl, Joao. 2007. *Will to Live. AIDS Therapies and the Politics of Survival.* Princeton: Princeton University Press.

———. 2014. "Ethnography in the Way of Theory." In *The Ground Between: Anthropologists Engage in Philosophy*, ed. Veena Das, Michael Jackson, and Arthur Kleinman, 94–118. Durham: Duke University Press.

Biehl, Joao, and Adriana Petryna. 2013. "Critical Global Health." In *When People Come First: Critical Studies in Global Health*, 1–23. Princeton: Princeton University Press.

Blomgren Maria, and Eva Sunden. 2008. "Constructing a European Healthcare Market: The Private Healthcare Company Capio and the Strategic Aspect of the Drove for Transparency." *Social Science & Medicine* 67, no. 10: 1512–20.

Bockman, Johanna. 2011. *Markets in the Name of Socialism: The Left-Wing Origins of Neoliberalism.* Stanford, CA: Stanford University Press.

Borneman, John. 1997. "Caring and Being Cared For: Displacing Marriage, Kinship, Gender and Sexuality." In *The Ethics of Kinship*, ed. James Faubion. Totowa, NJ: Rowland and Littlefield, 573–84.

Brotherton, Sean. 2012. *Revolutionary Medicine: Health and Body in Post-Soviet Cuba.* Durham: Duke University Press.

Buch, Elana D. 2014. "Troubling Gifts of Care: Vulnerable Persons and Threatening Exchanges in Chicago's Home Care Industry." *Medical Anthropology Quarterly* 28, no. 4: 599–615.

Burawoy, Michael, and Katherine Verdery. 1999. *Uncertain Transitions: Ethnographies of Change in the Postsocialist World*. New York: Rowman & Littlefield.

Burri, Regula, and Joseph Dumit, eds. 2007. *Biomedicine as Culture: Instrumental Practices, Technoscientific Knowledge, and New Modes of Life*. London: Routledge.

Byung-Chul, Han. 2015. *The Transparency Society*. Redwood City, CA: Stanford University Press.

Černiauskas, Gediminas. 1996. *Lietuvos Sveikatos Priežiūros Sistema Pereinamuoju laikotarpiu*. Vilnius: PHARE Sveikatos Priežiūros Reformos Projektas.

Clark, Adele E., Janet K. Clark, Janet Shim, Laura Mamo, and Jennifer K. Fishman. 2010. "Charting (Bio)medicine and (Bio) Medicalization: US Healthscapes and Iconography, 1890–Present." In *Biomedicalization, Technoscience and Illness in the U.S.*, 104–47. Durham: Duke University Press.

Clastres, Pierre. 1989. *Society against the State: Essays in Political Anthropology*. New York: Zone Books.

Cohen, Lawrence. 2008. "Politics of Care: Commentary on Janelle S. Taylor, 'On Recognition, Caring, and Dementia.'" *Medical Anthropology Quarterly*, 22, no. 4: 336–39.

Collier, Stephen J. 2011. *Post-Soviet Social: Neoliberalism, Social Modernity, Biopolitics*. Princeton: Princeton University Press.

Collier, Stephen, and Andrew Lakoff. 2005. "Regimes of Living." In *Global Assemblages: Technology, Politics, and Ethics as Anthropological Problems*, ed. Ahiwa Ong and Stephen J. Collier, 22–39. Malden, MA: Blackwell.

Cooper, Melinda. 2008. *Life as Surplus: Biotechnology and Capitalism in the Neoliberal Era*. Seattle: University of Washington Press.

de Certeau, Michel. 1984. *The Practice of Everyday Life*. Oakland: University of California Press.

de la Cadena, Marisol. 2015. *Earth Beings: Ecologies of Practice across Andean Worlds*. Durham: Duke University Press.

de la Cadena, Marisol, and Mario Blaser, eds. 2018. *A World of Many Worlds*. Durham: Duke University Press.

Delueze, Gilles, and Felix Guatarri. 2004. *A Thousand Plateaus: Capitalism and Schizophrenia*. London: Continuum.

Dao, Amy, and Jessica Mulligan. 2015. "Toward an Anthropology of Insurance and Health Reform: An Introduction to the Special Issue." *Medical Anthropology Quarterly* 30, no. 1: 5–17.

Das, Veena. 2006. *Life and Words: Violence and Decent into the Ordinary*. Berkeley: University of California Press.

Das, Veena, and Ranendra Das. 2007. "How the Body Speaks." In *Subjectivity: Ethnographic Investigations*, ed. Joao Biehl, Byron Good, and Arthur Kleinman, 66–97. Berkeley: University of California Press.

Das, Veena, and Clara Han. 2015. "A Concept Note." In *Living and Dying in the Contemporary World*, 1–38. Berkeley: University of California Press.

D'Avella, Nicholas. 2014. "Ecologies of Investment: Crisis Histories and Brick Futures in Argentina." *Cultural Anthropology* 29, no. 1: 173–99.

Day, Stephanie. 2015. "Waiting and the Architecture of Care." In *Living and Dying in the Contemporary World*, ed. Veena Das and Clara Han, 167–84. Berkeley: University of California Press.

DelVecchio Good, M. J., T. Munakata, Y. Kobayashi, C. Mattingly, C., and B. J. Good. 1994. "Oncology and Narrative Time." *Social Science and Medicine* 38, no. 6: 855–62.

Dodd, Nigel. 2014. *The Social Life of Money*. Princeton: Princeton University Press.

Drew, Jennifer, John D. Stoeckle, and Andrew J. Billings. 1983. "Tips, Status and Sacrifice: Gift Giving in the Doctor-Patient Relationship." *Social Science and Medicine* 17, no. 7: 99–404.

Dumit, Joseph. 2012. *Drugs for Life: How Pharmaceutical Companies Define Our Health*. Durham: Duke University Press.

Dunn, Elizabeth. 2004. *Privatizing Poland: Baby Food, Big Business, and the Remaking of Labor*. Ithaca, NY: Cornell University Press.

———. 2008. "Postsocialist Spores: Disease, Bodies, and the State in the Republic of Georgia." *American Ethnologist* 35, no. 2: 243–48.

Dzenovska, Dace. 2018. *The School of Europeanness: Tolerance or Other Lessons in Political Liberalism in Latvia*. Ithaca, NY: Cornell University Press.

Evans-Pritchard, E. E. 1976. *Witchcraft Oracles and Magic among the Azande*. Oxford: Clarendon Press.

Fassin, Didier. 2009. "Another Politics of Life Is Possible." *Theory, Culture & Society* 26, no. 5: 44–60.

Farmer, Paul. 1999. *Infections and Inequalities: The Modern Plagues*. Berkeley: University of California Press.

———. 2004. *Pathologies of Power: Health, Human Rights, and the New War on the Poor*. Berkeley: University of California Press.

Farquhar, Judith, and Lili Lai. 2015. "Nationality Medicines in China: Institutional Radionality and Healing Charisma." *Comparative Studies in Society and History* 57, no. 1: 381–406.

Farquhar, Judith, and Qicheng Zhang. 2012. *Ten Thousand Things: Nurturing Life in Contemporary China*. New York: Zone Books.

Favret-Saada, Jeanne. 1981. *Deadly Words: Witchcraft in the Bocage*. Cambridge: Cambridge University Press.

Ferguson, James. 2015. *Give a Man a Fish: Reflections on the New Politics of Distribution*. Durham: Duke University Press.

Field, Mark G. 1991. "The Hybrid Profession: Soviet Medicine." In *Professions and the States: Expertise and Autonomy in the Soviet Union and Eastern Europe*, ed. by Anthony Jones, 43–62. Philadelphia: Temple University Press.

Foucault, Michel. 1988. *The History of Sexuality*. Vol. 3: *The Care of the Self*. New York: Vintage Books.

———. 1990a. *The History of Sexuality*. Vol. 1: *An Introduction*. New York: Vintage Books.

———. 1990b. *The History of Sexuality*. Vol. 2: *The Use of Pleasure*. New York: Vintage Books.

———. 2008. *The Birth of Biopolitics: Lectures at the College de France, 1978–1979*. New York: Palgrave Macmillan.

Gaal, P., P.C. Belli, M. McKee, and M. Szócska. 2006. "Informal Payments for Health Care: Definitions, Distinctions, and Dilemmas." *Journal of Health Politics, Policy and Law* 31, no. 2: 251–93.

Garcia, Angela. 2010. *The Pastoral Clinic. Addiction and Dispossession along the Rio Grande*. Berkeley: University of California Press.

Giordano, Cristiana. 2014. *Migrants in Translation: Caring and the Logics of Difference in Contemporary Italy*. Berkeley: University of California Press.

Godbout, Jaques, and Alain Caille. 1998. *The World of the Gift*. Montreal: McGill-Queen's University Press.

Good, Byron J. 1994. *Medicine, Rationality and Experience: Anthropological Perspective*. Cambridge: Cambridge University Press.

Good, Byron J., and Mary-Jo DelVecchio Good. 1993. "'Learning Medicine': The Constructing of Medical Knowledge at Harvard Medical School." In *Knowledge, Power and Practice: The Anthropology of Medicine and Everyday Life*, ed. Shirley Lindenbaum and Margaret Lock, 81–107. Berkeley: University of California Press.

Graeber, David. 2011. *Debt: The First 5,000 Years*. Brooklyn: Melville House.

Gregory, C.A. 2015. *Gifts and Commodities*. 2nd ed. Chicago: HAU Books.

Greenhouse, Carol J. 2002. "Introduction: Altered States, Altered Lives." In *Ethnography in Unstable Places: Everyday Lives in Contexts of Dramatic Political Change*, 1–36. Durham: Duke University Press.

——, ed. 2012. *Ethnographies of Neoliberalism*. Philadelphia: University of Pennsylvania Press.

Gudžinskas, Liutauras. 2013. "Lietuvos ir Estijos Sveikatos Apsaugos Raida: Panašios Sąlygos, Skirtingi Rezultatai." *Politologija* 67, no. 3: 61–94.

Guyer, Jane. 1995. *Money Matters: Instability, Values, and Social Payments in the Modern African Communities*. Portsmouth, NH: Heinemann.

——. 2004. *Marginal Gains: Monetary Transactions in Atlantic Africa*. Chicago: University of Chicago Press.

——. 2009. "Composites, Fictions, and Risk: Toward an Ethnography of Price." In *Market and Society*, ed. Chris Han and Keith Hart, 203–21. Cambridge: Cambridge University Press.

——. 2012. "Soft Currencies, Cash Economies, New Monies: Past and Present." *Proceedings of the National Academy of Sciences* 109, no. 7: 2214–21.

Hahn, Robert A., and Arthur Kleinaman. 1983. "Belief as Pathogen, Belief as Medicine: 'Voodoo Death' and the 'Placebo Phenomenon' in Anthropological Perspective." *Medical Anthropology Quarterly* 14, no. 4: 3–19.

Hajekas, Fridrich, A. 1991. *Kelias į vergovę*. Vilnius: Mintis.

Haller, Dieter, and Cris Shore, eds. 2005. *Corruption: Anthropological Perspectives*. London: Pluto Press.

Han, Clara. 2012. *Life in Debt: Times of Care and Violence in Neoliberal Chile*. Berkeley: University of California Press.

Hann, Chris M., ed. 2002. *Postsocialism: Ideals, Ideologies and Practices in Eurasia*. Routledge.

Hart, Keith. 2001. *Money in an Unequal World: Keith Hart and His Memory Bank*. New York: Textere.

——. 2005. "Notes on towards an Anthropology of Money." *Kritikos* 2. https://intertheory.org/hart.htm.

Hart, Keith, and Horacio Ortiz. 2014. "The Anthropology of Money and Finance: Between Ethnography and World History." *Annual Review of Anthropology* 43: 465–82.

Hart, Keith, Jean-Louis Laville, and Antonio Cattani. 2010. *The Human Economy*. Cambridge: Polity Press.

Henare, Amiria, Martin Holbraad, and Sari Wastell, eds. 2007. *Thinking through Things: Theorising Artifacts Ethnographically*. London: Routledge.

Hetherington, Kregg. 2011. *Guerrilla Auditors: The Politics of Transparency in Neoliberal Paraguay*. Durham: Duke University Press.

Humphrey, Caroline. 2002. *The Unmaking of Soviet Life: Everyday Economies after Socialism*. Ithaca, NY: Cornell University Press.

——. 2012. "Favors and 'Normal Heroes': The Case of Postsocialist Higher Education." *HAU: Journal of Ethnographic Theory* 2, no. 2: 22–41.

Hunt, Lynda, Hannah S. Bell, Allison M. Baker, and Heather A. Howard. 2017. "Electronic Health Records and the Disappearing Patient." *Medical Anthropology Quarterly* 31, no. 3: 403–21.

Jackson, Michael. 2006. *The Politics of Storytelling: Violence, Transgression and Intersubjectivity*. Copenhagen: Museum Tusculanum Press.

Jankauskienė, Danguolė. 2000. *Sveikatos sistemos reformos Lietuvoje 1990–1998 įvertinimas. Daktaro disertacija (Biomedicinos mokslai, Visuomenės sveikata)*. Vilnius: Kauno medicinos universitetas.

Jasarevic, Larisa. 2016. *Health and Wealth on the Bosnian Market*. Bloomington: University of Indiana Press.

Kaufman, Sheron. 2015. *Ordinary Medicine: Extraordinary Treatments, Longer Lives, and Where to Draw the Line*. Durham: Duke University Press.

Keshavjee, Salmaan. 2014. *Blind Spot. How Neoliberalism Infiltrated Global Health*. Berkeley: University of California Press.

Kleinman, Arthur. 1988. *The Illness Narrative: Suffering, Healing & the Human Condition*. New York: Basic Books.

——. 2009. "The Art of Medicine. Caregiving: The Odyssey of Becoming More Human." *Lancet* 373, no. 24: 292–93.

Klumbyte, Neringa. 2011. "Political Intimacy: Power, Laughter, and Coexistence in Late Soviet Lithuania." *East European Politics and Societies* 25, no. 4: 658–77.

Knauss, William A. 1980. *Inside Russian Medicine: An American Doctor's First-Hand Report*. New York: Everest House.

Koch, Erin. 2013. *Free Market Tuberculosis: Managing Epidemics in Postsocialist Georgia*. Nashville: Vanderbilt University Press.

Kornai, Janos. 2000. "The Borderline between the Spheres of Authority of the Citizen and the State: Recommendations for the Hungarian Health Reform." In *Reforming the State. Fiscal and Welfare Reform in Post-Socialist Countries*, ed. J. Kornai, S. Haggard, and R. R. Kaufman, 181–219. Cambridge: Cambridge University Press.

Kornai, Janos, and Karen Eggleston. 2001. *Welfare, Choice, and Solidarity in Transition: Reforming the Health Sector in Eastern Europe*. Cambridge: Cambridge University Press.

Laville, Jean-Louis. 2010. "Plural Economy." In *The Human Economy*, ed. Keith Hart, Jean-Louis Laville, and Antonio Cattani, 77–83. Cambridge: Polity Press.

Ledeneva, Alena. 1998. *Russia's Economy of Favors: Blat, Networking and Informal Exchange*. Cambridge: Cambridge University Press.

——. 2000. "Continuity and Change of Blat Practices in Soviet and Post-Soviet Russia." In *Bribery and Blat in Russia: Negotiating Reciprocity from the Middle Ages to 1990s*, ed. Stephen Lovell, Alena Ledeneva, and A. S. Rogachevski, 183–205. New York: St. Martin's Press.

Lemon, Alaina. 1998. "'Your Eyes Are Green Like Dollars': Counterfeit Cash, National Substance, and Currency Apartheid in 1990s Russia." *Cultural Anthropology* 12, no. 1: 22–55.

Levi-Strauss, Claude. 1963. *Structural Anthropology*. New York: Basic Books.

——. 1976. *Structural Anthropology*. Vol. 2. Chicago: University of Chicago Press.

——. 1981. *The Naked Man*. New York: Harper and Row.

Likaitė, D., E. Čeponytė, and V. Nakrošis. 2015. "Asmens Sveikatos Proežiūros įstaigų tinklo restrktūrizavimas 2008–2012 metais: Kaip pavyko trečias etapas?" In *Kada reformos virsta pokyčiais? Politinis dėmesys, palaikymo koalicijos ir lyderystė A. Kubiliaus vyriausybės veiklos 2008–2012 metų laikotarpiu*, ed. V. Nakrošis, R. Barcevičius and R. Vilpišauskas, 189–250. Vilnius: Vilniaus Universiteto Leidykla.

Lock, Margaret, and Patricia Kaufert, eds. 1998. *Pragmatic Women and Body Politics*. New York: Cambridge University Press.

Lycklom, Laurie J. 1998. "Should Physicians Accept Gifts from Patients?" *JAMA*, December 9, 280, no. 22: 1944–46.

Malinowski, Bronislaw. [1922] 2010. *Argonauts of the Western Pacific*. Oxford: Benedicton Classics.

Martin, Emily. 2015. *The Meaning of Money in China and the United States*. Chicago: HAU Books.

Mattingly, Cheryl. 2012. *The Paradox of Hope: Journeys through a Clinical Borderland*. Berkeley: University of California Press.

Matza, Tomas. 2018. *Shock Therapy: Psychology, Precarity, and Well-Being in Postsocialist Russia*. Durham: Duke University Press.

Maurer, Bill. 2006. "Anthropology of Money." *Annual Review of Anthropology* 35: 15–36.

———. 2008. "Resocializing Finance? Or Dressing It in Mufti?" *Journal of Cultural Economy* 1, no. 1: 65–78.

———. 2012. "Payment: Forms and Functions of Value Transfer in Contemporary Society." *Cambridge Anthropology* 30, no. 2: 15–35.

Mauss, Marcel. [1950] 2001. *General Theory of Magic*. London: Routledge.

———. [1967] 2000. *The Gift: The Form and Reason of Exchange*. New York: Norton.

Merkšiūnaitė, Sandra. 2017. *Ligoninių veikla. Kaip atrodome Europos Sąjungoje? Visuomenės Sveikatos Netolygumai* 2, no. 21. Vilnius: Higienos Institutas. https://hi.lt/uploads/pdf/leidiniai/Informaciniai/VSNetolygumai%202017.2(21).pdf.

Miškinis, K., O. Riklikiene, R. Kalėdienė, and G. Jarašiūnaitė. 2011. "Lietuvos Gyventojų Informuotumas ir Pasitikėjimas Privalomojo Sveikatos Draudimo Sistema." *Sveikatos Mokslai* 21, no. 4: 48–61.

Moerman, Daniel. 2002. *Meaning, Medicine, and the "Placebo Effect."* Cambridge: Cambridge University Press.

Mol, Annemarie. 2002. *The Body Multiple*. London: Duke University Press.

———. 2008. *The Logic of Care: Health and the Problem of Patient Choice*. London: Routledge.

Mol, Annemarie, I. Moser, and J. Pols, eds. 2010. *Care in Practice: On Tinkering in Clinics, Homes and Farms*. Bielefeld: Transcript.

Morris, Jeremy, and Abel Polese. 2014. "Informal Health and Education Sector Payments in Russian and Ukrainian Cities: Structuring Welfare from Below." *European Urban and Regional Studies* 23, no. 3: 481–96.

Morris, Rosalind. 2004. "Intimacy and Corruption in Thailand's Age of Transparency." In *Off Stage/On Display: Intimacy and Ethnography in the Age of Public Culture*, 225–43. Stanford: Stanford University Press.

Murauskiene, Liubove. 2013. "Pacientų mokėjimų, sutikimo ir galimybių mokėti už sveikatos priežiūros paslaugas lygybės aspektai." *Sveikatos Politika ir Valdymas* 1, no. 5: 70–81.

Murauskiene, Liubove, Raimonda Janoniene, Marija Veniute, Ginneken van Ewout, and Marina Karanikolos. 2013. "Lithuania: Health System Review." *Health Systems in Transition* 15, no. 2: 1–150.

Narotzky, Susana, and Niko Bernier. 2014. "Crisis, Value, and Hope: Rethinking the Economy. An Introduction to Supplement." *Current Anthropology* 55, no. 9: 4–16.

Navarro, Vicente. 1977. *Social Security and Medicine in the USSR a Marxist Critique.* Lexington, MA: Lexington Books.

Norkus, Zenonas. 2014. *Du nepriklausomybės dvidešimtmečiai. Kapitalizmas, klasės ir demokratija Pirmojoje ir Antrojoje Lietuvos Respublikoje Lyginamosios Istorinės Sociologijos Požiūriu.* Vilnius: Aukso Žuvys.

Nuijten, Monique, and Gerhard Anders, eds. 2007. *Corruption and the Secret of Law: A Legal Anthropological Perspective.* London: Routledge.

Oliver, Adam. 2012. "Markets and Targets in the English National Health Service: Is There a Role for Behavioral Economics?" *Journal of Health Politics, Policy and Law* 37, no. 4: 647–64.

Ootes, S. T. C., A. J. Pols, E. H. Tonkens, and D. L. Willems. 2013. "Opening the Gift: Social Inclusion, Professional Codes and Gift-Giving in Long-Term Mental Healthcare." *Culture, Medicine and Psychiatry* 37: 131–47.

Ortner, Sherry B. 1973. "On Key Symbols." *American Anthropologist* 75, no. 5: 1338–46.

Patico, Jennifer. 2002. "Chocolate and Cognac: Gifts and the Recognition of Social Worlds in Post-Soviet Russia." *Ethnos* 67, no. 3: 345–68.

Parry, Jonathan, and Maurice Bloch, eds. 1989. *Money and Morality of Exchange.* Cambridge: Cambridge University Press.

Pedersen, Morten Axel, and Morten Nielsen. 2013. "Trans-Temporal Hinges: Reflections on a Comparative Ethnographic Study of Chinese Infrastructural Projects in Mozambique and Mongolia." *Social Analysis* 57, no. 1: 122–42.

Peebles Gustav. 2013. *The Euro and Its Rivals: Currency and the Construction of the International City.* Bloomington: Indiana University Press.

Petryna, Adriana. 2002. *Life Exposed: Biological Citizens After Chernobyl.* Princeton: Princeton University Press.

———. 2009. *When Experiments Travel: Clinical Trials and the Global Search for Human Subjects.* Princeton: Princeton University Press.

Philips, Sarah. 2011. *Disability and Mobile Citizenship in Postsocialist Ukraine.* Bloomington: Indiana University Press.

Pivorienė, J., and D. Mikalauskaitė. 2005. "Tarpukario Lietuvos socialinės apsaugos sistemos formavimosi prielaidos." *Socialinis darbas* 4, no. 1: 87–94.

Polese, Abel, and Jeremy Morris. 2014. *The Informal Post-Socialist Economy: Embedded Practices and Livelihoods.* London: Routledge.

Prentice, Rachel. 2013. *Bodies in Formation: An Ethnography of Anatomy and Surgery Education.* Durham: Duke University Press.

Puig de la Bellacasa, Maria. 2010. "Ethical Doings in Naturecultures: Ethics, Place and Environment." *Journal of Philosophy and Geography* 13, no. 2: 151–69.

Raikhel, Eugene. 2016. *Governing Habits: Treating Alcoholism in the Post-Soviet Clinic.* Ithaca, NY: Cornell University Press.

Ries, Nancy. 1997. *Russian Talk: Culture and Conversation during Perestroika.* Ithaca, NY: Cornell University Press.

Rivkin-Fish, Michelle. 2005. *Women's Health in Post-Soviet Russia: The Politics of Intervention.* Bloomington: Indiana University Press.

———. 2011. "Health, Gender, and Care Work: Productive Sites for Thinking Anthropologically about the Aftermaths of Socialism." *Anthropology of East Europe Review* 29, no. 1: 8–15.

Roberts, Bayard, Marina Karanikolos, and Bernd Rechel. 2014. "Health Trends." In *Trends in Health Systems in the Former Soviet Countries*, ed. B. Rechel, E.

Richardson, and M. McKee, 9–28. Observatory Studies Series 35. https://www.euro.who.int/__data/assets/pdf_file/0019/261271/Trends-in-health-systems-in-the-former-Soviet-countries.pdf.

Roberts, Elizabeth F. S. 2012. *God's Laboratory: Assisted Reproduction in the Andes*. Berkeley: University of California Press.

Roitman, Janet. 2004. *Fiscal Disobedience: An Anthropology of Economic Regulation in Central Africa*. Princeton: Princeton University Press.

Rose, Nikolas. 2007. *The Politics of Life Itself: Biomedicine, Power, and Subjectivity in the Twenty-First Century*. Princeton: Princeton University Press.

Rose, Nikolas, and Carlos Novas. 2005. "Biological Citizenship." In *Global Assemblages: Technology, Politics, and Ethics as Anthropological Problems*, ed. Ahiwa Ong and Stephen J. Collier, 439–63. Malden, MA: Blackwell.

Rutheford, Danilyn. 2001. "Intimacy and Alienation: Money and the Foreign in Biak." *Public Culture* 13, no. 2: 299–324.

Sachlins, Marshall David. 1974. *Stone Age Economics*. New Brunswick, NJ: Transaction Publishers.

Salmi, Anna-Maria. 2003. "Health in Exchange. Teachers, Doctors, and the Strength of Informal Practices in Russia." *Culture, Medicine, and Psychiatry* 27, no. 2: 109–30.

Sanders, Todd, and Harry G. West. 2003. "Power Revealed and Concealed in the New World Order, Transparency and Conspiracy." In *Ethnographies of Suspicion in the New World Order*, 1–37. Durham: Duke University Press.

Scheper-Hughes, Nancy. 1990. "Three Propositions for a Critically Applied Medical Anthropology." *Social Science and Medicine* 30, no. 2: 189–97.

Shell, Marc. 1995. *Art and Money*. Chicago: Chicago University Press.

Skultans, Veda. 2007. *Empathy and Healing: Essays in Medical and Narrative Anthropology*. New York: Berghahn Books.

Smart, Alan. 1993. "Gifts, Bribes and Guanxi: A Reconsideration of Bourdieu's Social Capital." *Cultural Anthropology* 8, no. 3: 388–408.

Stan, Sabina. 2007. "Transparency: Seeing, Counting and Experiencing the System." *Anthropologica* 49, no. 2: 257–73.

——. 2012. "Neither Commodities nor Gifts: Post-Socialist Informal Exchanges in the Romanian Healthcare system." *Journal of the Royal Anthropological Institute* 18, no. 1: 65–82.

Starkiene, Liudvika. 2012. "Gydytojų skaičiaus planavimas: Nuo mokslinių tyrimų iki sveikatos politikos." *Sveikatos politika ir valdymas: Mokslo darbai / Mykolo Romerio universitetas*. 1, no. 4: 102–15.

Stevenson, Lisa. 2012. "The Psychic Life of Biopolitics: Survival, Cooperation, and Inuit Community." *American Anthropologist* 39, no. 3: 592–613.

——. 2014. *Life Beside Itself: Imagining Care in the Canadian Arctic*. Berkeley: University of California Press.

Stewart, Kathleen. 1996. *A Space on the Side of the Road*. Princeton: Princeton University Press.

——. 2007. *Ordinary Affects*. London: Duke University Press.

Strassler, Karen. 2009. "The Face of Money: Currency, Crisis, and Remediation in Post-Suharto Indonesia" *Cultural Anthropology* 24, no. 1: 68–103.

Strathern, Marilyn. 1995. *The Relation: Issues in Complexity and Scale*. Cambridge: Prickly Pear Press.

——. 2000a. *Audit Cultures: Anthropological Studies in Accountability, Ethics, and the Academy*. London: Routledge.

———. 2000b. "The Tyranny of Transparency." *British Educational Research Journal* 26, no. 3: 309–21.

———. 2005. *Partial Connections*. Lanham, MD: Alta Mira Press.

———. 2020. *Relations: An Anthropological Account*. London: Duke University Press.

Sunder Rajan, Kaushik. 2006. *Biocapital: The Constitution of Postgenomic Life*. London: Duke University Press.

Taljūnaite, Meilute. 2012. "Gydytojų karjerą stabilizuonatys veiksniai." *Filosofija Sociologija* 23, no. 2: 154–63.

Taussig, Michael T. 1980. "Reification and the Consciousness of the Patient." *Social Science & Medicine* 14B: 3–13.

Taylor, Janelle. 2008. "On Recognition, Caring and Dementia." *Medical Anthropology Quarterly* 22, no. 4: 313–35.

Ticktin, Miriam. 2006. "Where Ethic and Politics Meet: The Violence of Humanitarianism in France." *American Ethnologist* 33, no. 1: 33–49.

———. 2011. *Casualties of Care: Immigration and the Politics of Humanitarianism in France*. Berkeley: University of California Press.

Transparency International. 2006. *Global Corruption Report: Corruption and Health*. https://www.transparency.org/en/publications/ global-corruption-report-2006-corruption-and-health.

Tronto, Joan C.1993. *Moral Boundaries: A Political Argument for an Ethic of Care*. New York: Routledge.

Tsing, Anna. 2005. *Friction: An Ethnography of Global Connection*. Princeton: Princeton University Press.

———. 2013. "Sorting Out Commodities: How Capitalist Value Is Made through Gifts." *HAU: Journal of Ethnographic Theory* 3, no. 1: 21–43.

———. 2015. *The Mushroom at the End of the World: On the Possibility of Life in Capitalist Ruins*. Princeton: Princeton University Press.

Twigg, Judyth L.2000. "Unfulfilled Hopes: The Struggle to Reform Russian Health Care and Its Financing." In *Russia's Torn Safety Nets: Health and Social Welfare during the Transition*, ed. Mark G. Field and J. L. Twigg, 43–64. New York: St. Martin's Press.

Vaiseta, Tomas. 2015. "Sovietinės sveikatos apsaugos sistemos diegimo atspindys gyventojų skunduose (1944–1953)." *Genocidas ir rezistencija* 1, no. 3: 51–62.

Verdery, Katherine. 1996. *What Was Socialism and What Comes After?* Princeton: Princeton University Press.

Verran, Helen. 2001. *Science and an African Logic*. Chicago: University of Chicago Press.

Waldby, Catherine, and Melinda Cooper. 2008. "The Biopolitics of Reproduction." *Australian Feminist Studies* 23, no. 5: 55–73.

Webb, Martin. 2012. "Activating Citizens, Remaking Brokerage: Transparency, Activism, Ethical Scenes, and the Urban Poor in Dehli." *PoLAR* 35, no. 2: 206–22.

Whitmarsh, Ian. 2014. "The No/Name of the Institution." *Anthropological Quarterly* 87, no. 3: 855–82.

Yang, Mayfair Mei-Hui. 1994. *Gifts, Favors, and Banquets: The Art of Social Relationships in China*. Ithaca, NY: Cornell University Press.

Young, Alan. 1982. "The Anthropologies of Illness and Sickness" *Annual Review of Anthropology* 11: 257–85.

Yurchak, Alexei. 2002. "Entrepreneurial Governmentality in Post-Socialist Russia: A Cultural Investigation of Business Practices." In *The New Entrepreneurs of*

Europe and Asia, ed. V. E. Bonnell and T. B. Gold, 278–322. Armonk, NY: M.E. Sharpe.

——. 2003. "Russian Neoliberal: The Enterpreneural Ethic and the Spirit of 'True Careerism.'" *Russian Review* 62, no. 1: 72–90.

———. 2006. *Everything Was Forever, Until It Was No More: The Last Soviet Generation*. Princeton: Princeton University Press.

Zaloom, Caitlin. 2003. "Ambiguous Numbers: Trading Technologies and Interpretation in Financial Markets." *American Ethnologist* 30, no. 2: 258–72.

Zelizer, Viviana.1997. *The Social Meaning of Money*. Princeton: Princeton University Press.

Zhang, Li, and Aihwa Ong, eds. 2008. *Privatizing China: Socialism from Afar*. Ithaca, NY: Cornell University Press.

Zigon, Jarret. 2011. *"HIV Is God's Blessing": Rehabilitating Morality in Neoliberal Russia*. Berkeley: University of California Press.

Index

Page numbers in *italics* refer to figures.

CPSIA information can be obtained
at www.ICGtesting.com
Printed in the USA
JSHW022317240523
42204JS00003B/69